The Essential Guide to Intermittent Fasting for Women

Megan Ramos is a clinical educator, researcher, and co-founder, with Dr Jason Fung, of 'The Fasting Method'. After losing 86 pounds and reversing her own metabolic conditions, she has become a world-leading expert on therapeutic fasting and low-carbohydrate diets and has guided thousands of people worldwide to weight loss and better health. She is a co-author of the *New York Times* best-seller *Life in the Fasting Lane*.

The Essential Guide to Intermittent Fasting for Women

balance your hormones to lose weight, lower stress, and optimise health

MEGAN RAMOS

Foreword by **Dr Jason Fung**

SCRIBE

Melbourne • London

Scribe Publications
18–20 Edward St, Brunswick, Victoria 3056, Australia
2 John St, Clerkenwell, London, WC1N 2ES, United Kingdom
3754 Pleasant Ave, Suite 100, Minneapolis, Minnesota 55409, USA

First Published by Greystone Books Ltd.
343 Railway Street, Suite 302, Vancouver, B.C. V6A 1A4, Canada
Published by Scribe 2023
Reprinted 2024

Internal pages designed by Fiona Siu

Printed and bound in Australia by Griffin Press

Scribe is committed to the sustainable use of natural resources and the use of paper products made responsibly from those resources.

Scribe acknowledges Australia's First Nations peoples as the traditional owners and custodians of this country, and we pay our respects to their elders, past and present.

978 1 761380 26 6 (paperback)
978 1 761385 06 3 (ebook)

Catalogue records for this book are available from the National Library of Australia.

scribepublications.com.au
scribepublications.co.uk
scribepublications.com

Contents

Foreword

INTERMITTENT FASTING HAS become one of the hottest topics in weight loss, both in the public eye and in academic medicine, for a good reason: it works. If you don't eat, generally you'll lose weight. Megan Ramos is one of the pioneers in the use of intermittent fasting for weight loss, and we worked together in the early years of fasting's renaissance in the mid-2010s to promote this ancient, time-tested practice.

Megan had suffered, like many others, from weight gain and polycystic ovary syndrome. As the years went on, her weight became harder to control. Despite rigorously following the standard nutritional advice of the day and receiving expensive private dietary counseling from some of the most prominent dieticians, Megan only got sicker. Thanks to her knowledge as a medical researcher, she could sense something was amiss.

I am a physician, a nephrologist (kidney specialist) by training. With the ongoing epidemic of type 2 diabetes, kidney disease was increasing steadily. Diabetes had become—and is still—the single most common cause of kidney disease (along with blindness, infections, and nontraumatic amputations). Standard medical treatment was not helping, and I gradually recognized that we were largely ignoring the root cause of the problem.

Weight gain and obesity were driving the epidemic of diabetes. Therefore, for people to get better, the solution was not medications but weight loss. If people could lose weight, then their type 2 diabetes would improve. If they didn't have diabetes, they would not develop diabetic kidney disease. Prevention was much better than treatment. But the mainstay of standard diabetes treatment focused on prescribing medications to reduce blood glucose, instead of changing people's diets and lifestyles.

As I researched weight loss, I considered the use of fasting as a therapeutic tool. Megan, a researcher I was working with, became immediately fascinated. This idea, we felt, was worth investigating further. In the early 2010s, fasting was considered a dangerous practice. People were convinced that eating six or even ten times a day was healthy. The very idea of not eating for a period of time was widely acknowledged as risky. But why?

The science behind fasting is clear: there is nothing inherently unusual or dangerous about it. Fasting is simply the period of time that you do not eat. There is a balance between feeding (when you store food energy or calories) and fasting (when you burn calories). Fasting allows the body to use its own stores of food energy: body fat. Fasting is natural and traditional, and more importantly, it works to reduce weight and reverse type 2 diabetes. Many of the myths and negative beliefs around fasting have proven to be untrue.

Megan and I started the Intensive Dietary Management clinic to put some of these ideas into practice, and we saw the health results immediately. Some of our patients' stories were unbelievable. After years of disease, they were losing weight, reducing their type 2 diabetic medications, and just getting better. It's been a long road, but fasting is once again regaining acceptance. Megan has been at the forefront of this movement, especially for women, and this book of science-based advice and practical tips will prove to be a valuable resource for many years to come.

DR. JASON FUNG, author of *The Obesity Code* and *The Diabetes Code*

Introduction

• • • • •

"One cannot think well, love well,
sleep well, if one has not dined well."

VIRGINIA WOOLF

M Y NAME IS Megan Ramos, and I'm a clinical educator and researcher who specializes in using intermittent fasting to help prevent, heal, and reverse chronic health conditions such as obesity and type 2 diabetes. I've provided fasting and nutrition education and coaching for thousands of people with metabolic syndrome.

Eating in timed windows that change from day to day, which is essentially what intermittent fasting is, is significantly easier than radically changing my diet, in my experience. Maintaining a regular schedule of intermittent fasting has been transformative to my life. Over the years, I've discovered that intermittent fasting has addressed the root causes of my poor health while giving me the freedom to eat all kinds of meat, poultry, fish, and vegetables, with the occasional treat thrown in!

As we'll explore in this book, intermittent fasting is a way to reduce the number of hours you consume food so that your body can rebalance its hormones and you can gain control of your health. I encourage you to read each chapter without skipping ahead so that you understand how the body works, how to support your health, and how to find a fasting schedule that suits your lifestyle and helps address the root causes of your own health challenges. I know it's tempting to jump ahead—that's exactly what I would want to do too.

I want this book to be both educative and personal. I have been through my own health struggles and benefited personally from intermittent fasting during my journey to wellness. When you see the changes I've made in my own life and read the stories of other women who have healed from chronic illness and other health challenges, I hope you'll find inspiration and resources to make intermittent fasting part of your journey to wellness too. I've made it easy for you to incorporate intermittent fasting into your life if you follow along step by step.

I wrote this book for you and for all women, young and old. I've spent my whole life thinking about how we, as women, can help ourselves be healthier, and I want to share everything I know with you.

My Journey to Intermittent Fasting

I was born in 1984, a time when many real, whole foods were labeled as "bad." In March of that year, *Time* magazine featured a photo of bacon and eggs on its front cover under the title "Cholesterol: And Now the Bad News...," and those foods certainly weren't allowed in my home. My parents were busy, so if I didn't like what was being cooked for dinner, I'd just order pizza.

But my journey to this career and this life really began during my preteen years when my mother became very sick. She was diagnosed with a rare genetic condition called neurofibromatosis type 2, which means her body grows benign tumors on her central nervous system. She also has several clusters of brain tumors called meningiomas. And her body grows benign endocrine tumors as well. No one's sure why. As a result, she had a tumor removed from the middle of her spinal cord, and she's had her thyroid gland removed along with one of her adrenal glands. In fact, the tumor on her adrenal gland was so substantial that it caused her body to produce excess cortisol, our primary stress hormone (see Chapter 5).

The wild hormonal fluctuations from these endocrine tumors caused my mom's hip to fracture. No fall. No accident. Nothing. She just lost the ability to walk, and because this symptom was so unusual, it took doctors six months to diagnose what was happening. Even at the time, it seemed to me that there must be a root cause to my mom's condition—and that doctors were missing it.

I became angry. Accepting that a healthy woman suddenly became sick and not trying to understand *why* seemed wrong. I wanted doctors to be delving into the causes of her illness, not just prescribing solutions that failed to work. The more I thought about it, the more enraged I became. Someone needed to solve this problem, and in tenth grade I decided that someone was going to be me.

The following summer, I had the opportunity to work at a nephrology clinic in Toronto, Canada. Not only was this kidney clinic part of the largest medical program of any kind in North America, but they also did a lot of research. They did pharmaceutical research and research focused on earlier diagnosis of kidney disease, and they were also interested in lifestyle interventions. From day one, I was allowed to interact with patients and learn about their diseases, medications, and lifestyles. I returned to the clinic every summer through high school; when I started university, I continued to work there part-time. I loved the work, and my favorite moments were connecting with patients. Many of them watched me grow up. They stopped being only patients to me. They were friends, and in some cases, they became family.

Life expectancy on dialysis is three years if you have diabetes and five years if you don't. The worst part of the job was when one of these people passed. My heart shattered every time an obituary was passed around. And that solidified my desire to find sustainable solutions that would transform people's lives. But as the years went by, I lost hope that the work could make a difference. Too many people were dying, mostly from type 2 diabetes and obesity. Nothing the clinic recommended was helping. I felt as powerless as I had when my mom got ill; all I was discovering with my career was *when* people were going to die, not how to help them get better.

When I was twenty-six, I took a year off school. I needed time to think about what I was going to do with my life. I wanted to help people, but all I was doing was watching the people I'd grown to love die. My passion for the work cooled, and I became clinical because it was easier to avoid getting attached to my patients, to accept that I couldn't do anything to help them. I applied to study actuarial science—I certainly didn't have to worry about people breaking my heart in that profession. I was desperate to find my calling since medicine didn't appear to be it.

I also felt hopeless about my future. Obesity, type 2 diabetes, and heart disease ran in my family. And my mother was still suffering in baffling ways. This genetic heritage made me concerned not only for my mother's health but also for my own. Despite being what my girlfriends called "obnoxiously skinny," I had two diseases associated with obesity: nonalcoholic fatty liver disease (NAFLD) and polycystic ovary syndrome (PCOS). No one had explained *why* I had these diseases. In hindsight, I realize it's because I had such a high percentage of body fat, but doctors are poorly educated on obesity, so no one offered me any helpful insights. I was told I'd grow out of these conditions as I got older so long as I stayed "skinny."

I stayed skinny, but the fatty liver, PCOS, and fatigue seemed to get worse, and I began to feel hopeless and depressed.

I realized that I had to take control of my own health. I wanted to start eating like a responsible adult. I made a promise to myself that twenty-six was going to be my year of finally directing my career and my personal health. Following Canada's Food Guide, I began to eat six small meals a day. That meant eating lots of snacks, counting my calories, limiting my fat intake, and boosting my intake of "healthy" whole grains and fruits. I worked out with a personal trainer.

You name it, I did it.

I gained 80 pounds.

Years of poor eating habits led me to the doctor's office around the time of my twenty-seventh birthday.

"I'm afraid to say that you have type 2 diabetes," the doctor announced once she'd reviewed my bloodwork. I thought I'd misheard. I knew the outcomes for people with type 2 diabetes; I saw those outcomes all the time at the nephrology clinic where I worked. I pictured the patients I'd lost, and my heart sank. My eyes welled up with tears. The adrenaline pumped through my veins. I was utterly terrified.

I was twenty-seven, and I was broken. What kind of life was I going to have? I pictured kidney failure by age thirty-five, blindness by forty, dementia or Alzheimer's by fifty. At some point, cancer would get me. I called in sick to work that afternoon and cried. I believed there was nothing that doctors could offer me. There were no answers, no solutions, no understanding of what was happening to my body, or to the bodies of so many women I knew. Like so many others, I was expected to function with a sick body, a terrified heart, and a broken mind. I didn't tell anyone about my diabetes, but I started to live like I was dying.

My Recovery With Intermittent Fasting

A few weeks after my diagnosis, a colleague came into our research office and said, "You won't believe this! Dr. Fung thinks you can cure people of type 2 diabetes through starvation. I think he's losing it!"

At the time, Dr. Jason Fung was one of the youngest nephrologists on the team. He was exceptionally well read, and he often presented ideas that were outside of the box but made a lot of sense. I remember feeling very uncomfortable about my colleague's laughter, but I was too unwell to really process what she was saying and I didn't follow up.

A couple of weeks later, I was reviewing some lab results in the back of the office one afternoon, and I overheard Dr. Fung giving a presentation nearby. I popped into the presentation room and found him talking to a group of patients about intermittent fasting for type 2 diabetes reversal and sustainable weight loss. I knew that Dr. Fung, like me, was frustrated that so many of his patients were suffering in such poor health. They were getting sick, and every day he was delivering bad news. He'd been researching diabetes and exploring an avenue connecting religion, fasting, spirituality, and health. Everything he said that day was contradictory to what I'd been taught and to how doctors practice medicine—but all of it made sense based on my clinical experience. It was like a key fitting into a lock: a new door was opened for me.

I rushed home after the presentation to scour the internet for information about fasting. I read that intermittent fasting was a way of controlling when I ate food and that by fasting I could transform my health. I decided to dive in and take control of my roster of diseases. The next day, I elected to fast for seven days . . . and I made it about seventeen hours before I was ready to eat the drywall in the office.

What I did when I first started is a cautionary tale, and certainly not how I recommend you begin your own path to intermittent fasting. Jumping headlong into fasting can lead you to become dispirited and frustrated with the process, and it can be dangerous for some people. I quickly learned that I needed to take a flexible, gradual approach, which as a perfectionist and extremist was hard for me to understand. But that's the approach that I'm here to help you learn. I've experienced this approach firsthand, and I've helped guide thousands of clients on their own fasting journeys, honing and shaping the method for each individual.

After my initial failure, I did more research and decided to skip breakfast for a few days in a row. It seemed easy because I had no time to eat breakfast anyway. I also elected to avoid snacking between lunch and dinner. I told myself I needed to treat fasting not as a diet but as a therapeutic treatment. My goal initially wasn't to lose weight; it was to reverse my type 2 diabetes. And so I showed up to every fasting day like I would have for chemotherapy. Fasting was my treatment.

Fasting was tough at first, but it got easier over the weeks and months that followed. As I started to feel better, I found I had the energy to eat better. I could actually stand in the kitchen after work and cook a meal without falling over. Within six months, I reversed my type 2 diabetes, PCOS, and fatty liver, and I lost just over 60 pounds. My periods became regular for the first time in my life. And flash forward: I'm still free of all my medical conditions and have maintained an 86-pound weight loss for the last ten years.

Sharing the Message of Intermittent Fasting

Shortly after my initial success with fasting, Dr. Fung and I joined forces to start some nephrology patients with type 2 diabetes on a fasting program. Within a matter of weeks, *all of them had eliminated at least one diabetic medication, if not all their diabetic medications*. And people of all ages were suddenly losing weight, even when they thought they couldn't lose 50, 70, or 100 pounds at their advanced ages. Our colleagues were astounded by what we were doing, and they started to refer patients to us. Soon news spread in the community, and before we knew it, we had a two-year waitlist for the clinic, which we initially called the Intensive Dietary Management (IDM) clinic.

Dr. Fung went on to author his first book, *The Obesity Code*, which instantly became an international bestseller in 2016. Within a month of the book's release, my email inbox was full of messages from people from all over the world begging to come to our clinic. We were overwhelmed. We didn't have the space to see everyone in person, and so I began to educate people online about fasting. The next thing I knew, I was working fourteen-hour days, seven days a week.

Today we operate the fasting program entirely online through a self-guided program with community support, health coaching, and telemedicine. To date, I've helped over 20,000 people worldwide regain control of their health and waistline through the power of intermittent fasting. Most of the people I've served are cisgender women. Young women with PCOS, which sometimes causes infertility. Women after they've finished having kids. Women entering menopause. Women going through menopause. Women who are postmenopausal. Fasting hasn't just helped these women: it's transformed their lives.

In this book, I'll guide you through the science and my clinical experience working with women from all stages of life, whose health concerns range from obesity to autoimmune conditions to type 2 diabetes, to help you discover how to heal. This knowledge is also helpful for women who want to maintain optimal weight and follow a preventive approach to caring for their future body. Often women are told that it's normal to gain weight and to get sick as we age. It's not true. You can take back control.

Fasting is an excellent way to benefit us all by keeping inflammation levels low, maintaining healthy weight, and preventing possible future health challenges. This book dispels the myths about fasting, fat, and food that so many women have been subjected to. It explores the complex hormones that women have and why these impact health and wellness, and it shows you how to use the power of intermittent fasting protocols to transform your health and your future.

In the past decade since Dr. Fung and I started IDM, intermittent fasting has become much better understood. Major news outlets, like CNN and *Time* magazine, cover fasting almost every day. I overhear young healthy-looking people talking about the benefits of fasting as I'm walking down the street. I see the positive impact of fasting on thousands of clients, and I want that same result for you. I have lots of clinical evidence, medical knowledge, and personal experience to share about intermittent fasting that can help you understand how our bodies work, resolve the root causes of illness, prevent disease, and achieve your healthiest body.

PART ONE

The Roots of Our Resistance:
Myths and Misunderstandings About Fasting, Fat, and Food

The Benefits and Myths of Intermittent Fasting for Women

. . . . . .

*"Our food should be our medicine.
Our medicine should be our food.
But to eat when you are sick is to feed your sickness."*
ATTRIBUTED TO HIPPOCRATES

NTERMITTENT FASTING (IF) is a simple, easy way to help you manage your weight, balance your hormones, and maintain a healthy body. Although IF has a reputation for being a new and trendy way to eat, it is in fact an age-old way of eating that will feel natural to you once you bring it into your life.

When I first heard of IF, I was so excited to get started that I made myself terribly hungry and almost gave up. If I hadn't been connected to people who were researching IF and understood how and why IF makes sense, I may never have progressed on this journey. So, I want to start by sharing information about what IF is—and what it is not—and some of the benefits of incorporating this eating and healing practice into your life. By sharing everything

I know, I'll help you build a solid foundation so you can make significant changes easily. I'll give you tools to succeed in your first fast, and every fast after that one—tools I've learned from my personal experiences and from my professional experiences working with thousands of others who've begun IF for the first time. We'll get to that part of the book shortly, but first let's begin by looking at some terms, including what we mean when we talk about fasting.

What Is Intermittent Fasting?

Fasting is one of the oldest ways of eating known to humans. Yet in 2013 when Dr. Jason Fung and I were trying to introduce fasting methods to our patients, we were met with a lot of mixed feedback from our colleagues. This is because when people hear the word *fasting*, they think *starvation*. The two words are actually opposites.

Fasting is the voluntary restriction of food for religious, spiritual, or health benefits. In contrast, *starvation* is the involuntary restriction of food. Starvation is not a choice, and it's not deliberate. When you choose to fast, food is available; it's that you choose not to eat it for a period of time. Here is an analogy.

A freezer stores food in the long term, and a refrigerator is used for short-term storage. Suppose that three times a day, every day, we go to the market to buy food. Some goes into the refrigerator, but the excess goes into the freezer. Soon one freezer is not enough, so we buy another, then another. Over a period of decades, we have ten freezers and nowhere else to put them. Food in the freezer does not get eaten because, three times a day, we still buy more food. There is simply no reason to release the food from the freezer.

What would happen if, one day, we decided not to buy food? Would everything shut down in "starvation mode"? Nothing could be further from the truth. We would first empty the refrigerator. Then the food, so carefully stored in the freezer, would be released.

— DR. JASON FUNG

This analogy shows how fasting and starvation are different: the freezer of our bodies has food in it, and when we fast, we use that fuel up. When we are starving, there is no food in the fridge or freezer, and we cannot find any fuel for our bodies.

At our clinic in Toronto, a lot of my patients were already comfortable with the idea of fasting because they fast for religious reasons. Or if they didn't fast themselves, they knew someone who did. When we talked about fasting three times a week, many of those patients understood it was manageable. Maybe you have experience of fasting because of your spiritual beliefs, or maybe the whole idea is very new to you. Either way, the word *fasting* refers to a number of different practices. I want to clearly explain the definitions I use in my clinical practice for different types of fast.

Finding the type of fast that suits you and your body is what I want to help you discover. Most importantly, I want you to find a path that you can maintain because **consistency is key in a journey to wellness.**

• THE LANGUAGE OF FASTING •

Intermittent fasting, also known as alternate-day fasting, is when you alternate times when you eat with times when you don't eat. The key is *intermittently*, which means that you fast often but not continuously or in the same way day in, day out. For example, I fast for 24 hours, three times each week. I time my own three fasts for Mondays, Wednesdays, and Fridays. This way the weekends are open to enjoy food with my husband. For most people to see consistent progress, fasting for 24 hours three times a week is the most helpful intermittent fasting program for losing weight, balancing hormones, and preventing and reversing type 2 diabetes and other insulin-related diseases.

Time-restricted eating is when you allow yourself to eat only between certain hours of each day. For example, you might find that 16 hours between the last time you eat in the evening (early supper) and the first time you eat in the morning (breakfast) is a time restriction that is manageable for you. That means from supper until a late breakfast, you don't consume food. Our first meal of the day is called *break-fast* for a reason! Often, people who are new to fasting begin with time-restricted eating, with great results.

One example of a time-restricted eating fast is a 16/8 fast. This means that you eat only during an 8-hour window. For 16 hours of the day, you do not consume food. Another common example is an 18/6 fast. Most people who do an 18/6 fast skip one meal a day, perhaps breakfast or supper. You eat during a 6-hour window, and there are 18 hours in the day when you are not eating.

These eating plans are not intermittent because they are followed every day in the same way. They're also not therapeutic fasting plans, because while they're great for maintaining good health, they're not great for weight loss for women with insulin-related issues. Insulin levels are not suppressed long enough for time-restricted eating to be a true intermittent fast, which makes it difficult to lose weight using this method. However, even a short break from eating can be beneficial. To make these eating plans intermittent, you need to change your eating schedule so that they are not the same pattern day in and day out. For example, you can do a 16/8 fast one day and follow it with a normal eating day. For best results, I recommend time-restricted eating for my clients on the days when they are not fasting.

Extended or *prolonged fasting* is any fast longer than 72 hours. Longer fasts can be great for a hormonal reset and for anti-aging but *they are not suitable for everyone*, and you shouldn't do them all the time or even that often. I recommend doing an extended fast *only with medical support* and with at least a six-to-eight-week gap between fasts. Too many extended fasts can cause fasting burnout, deep frustration, and nutrient deficiencies—especially vitamins D, K, and selenium. Selenium is essential for our thyroid function, and too little can lead to muscle weakness and fatigue. Too much selenium can have detrimental effects, too, and so people shouldn't go out and take lots of selenium to get them through prolonged fasting.

Angela's Story

During the COVID-19 pandemic lockdowns, Angela gained 20 pounds—as many people did. She told me that she's the sort of person who either goes to the gym seven days a week or doesn't go at all: an all-or-nothing personality type.

She'd turned to fasting to try to lose the weight she'd gained from constant snacking through those long pandemic days and nights at home. We'll learn in this book that constant snacking leads to chronic insulin secretion, which leads to weight gain.

The problem for Angela is that with fasting, she had tried the same all-or-nothing approach that she took to exercise: she was doing repeated five-day fasts to try to lose those 20 pounds. Doing back-to-back extended fasts led her to fasting fatigue, dehydration, and difficulty resisting foods because of a feeling of deprivation. This meant that she ate a lot and felt frustrated. She came to me looking for help.

In his book *Atomic Habits*, James Clear says that it's important to get 1 percent better over and over, and this was my advice to Angela: fast twice a week for 42 hours—and eat lunch and dinner without snacking on the other days. I really emphasized consistency, which, as you'll see, is key to my teachings.

Angela finally resigned to fasting twice a week, which suited her lifestyle better. Within six weeks, she was able to lose half her excess weight. As we'll explore often in this book, fasting consistently is far more powerful than extreme fasting to get results. Although we might think that if one day is good for us, ten days is better, this more is better approach is not sustainable or successful. Intermittent fasting provides many long-term benefits for women, and these benefits are maximized when IF is maintained consistently over a long period.

The Benefits of Intermittent Fasting for Women

Many women come to me with a specific reason to try fasting: they want to lose weight, increase their fertility, manage their type 2 diabetes, or find a sustainable way of eating that they can incorporate into their lives. Intermittent fasting addresses all of these issues and also benefits most adult women, no matter their current health or stage of life. There are many benefits to intermittent fasting: everything from maintaining weight loss to the incredible flexibility of this way of eating.

Maintains weight loss

When I first began to fast intermittently, I lost 60 pounds. And I've maintained an 86-pound weight loss for ten years through intermittent fasting. I've seen this sustained long-term weight loss time and time again, for thousands of my clients. I'll explore the reasons why IF leads to weight loss in Chapter 4, but weight loss is one of its primary benefits.

Reverses type 2 diabetes

When we eat sugar or starch, our blood sugar (glucose) levels naturally go up. Our blood sugar levels should decrease within two hours of eating, but if you have type 2 diabetes, those levels stay high. Intermittent fasting treats the root cause of type 2 diabetes, and the result is that you have a normal glucose response two hours after eating. We explore this response in more detail in Chapter 3.

Reverses polycystic ovary syndrome

PCOS is a disorder named for the fluid-filled growths that can develop on your ovaries. Depending on how many and how big these growths are, they can disrupt the sex hormones that are produced in your ovaries. These disruptions can lead to irregular menstrual cycles, infertility, obesity, and acne or facial hair growth.

Intermittent fasting is counter to growth, and so we see these growths go away because we're addressing the root cause. We'll look at PCOS in more detail in Chapter 7.

Reverses nonalcoholic fatty liver disease

NAFLD occurs when the liver accumulates so much fat that it can no longer function properly. This type of fat is visceral (it is located on our internal organs), and it causes disease. The liver controls whether our bodies can manage glucose efficiently, which is the same problem we see with type 2 diabetes. If we have problems with the liver, we have problems with type 2 diabetes. IF gives the body the chance to use this visceral fat as fuel, which helps to reverse NAFLD.

Lowers cholesterol

High levels of certain types of fats called cholesterols can increase our risk of heart disease and stroke. They can also exacerbate type 2 diabetes. Intermittent fasting reduces inflammation in the body, which reduces cholesterol levels.

Lowers blood pressure

High blood pressure levels create a heavy workload for your heart. When you fast intermittently, you lose excess water and sodium, and then your blood pressure comes down. How and why intermittent fasting helps lower blood pressure is a very large topic, beyond the scope of this book, but it's useful to know about this benefit as many women struggle with high blood pressure. High blood pressure is in fact a symptom of hyperinsulinemia—too much sugar and therefore insulin—and as you'll see throughout this book, fasting helps you lower your insulin levels. In turn, your blood pressure, if high, will lower.

Induces autophagy to prevent disease and slow aging

Autophagy is a physiological process in which the body hunts down broken and old cells and proteins, breaks them apart, and uses them to put together new healthy cells and proteins. When you are in a state of autophagy, your body is actively preventing disease and slowing aging. In Chapter 10, we look at how IF induces autophagy.

Makes scheduling simple and flexible for busy women

For me, one of the greatest benefits of intermittent fasting is how easy it is to schedule into my life. Women have to juggle so much. With IF, I don't have to be thinking about and planning meals all the time. On fasting days, I don't have to cook for myself at all, and I can put in a full workday and use my lunch break for a walk and stress relief, instead of trying to squeeze in a meal. I also value how easily I can select fasting days and eating days so I can allow for cake on my birthday or wonderful holiday meals with family and friends. In addition to IF's health benefits, its simplicity has helped me stay consistent in my eating habits. For more on IF and scheduling, see Chapter 10.

Despite all these very real, very tangible benefits, social media is plagued with posts saying that fasting is dangerous or does not work for women. In my personal and clinical experience, I have not seen anything but the amazing impact intermittent fasting, as well as time-restricted eating protocols, have on women at any stage of their lives. Throughout the book, I share my own experiences and those of clients, and I share research that shows how IF is effective for women.

As a scientist, I believe that it is always important to question what we're told. For example, I always tell my patients that my goal is for them to decide to fast because they understand why they are fasting and how it benefits them. I never want someone to fast on a Monday because Megan said they should. You should be fasting because you think the science behind it makes sense for you. So, let's break down some of the myths about fasting.

Fact or Fiction? Some Common Myths About Women and Fasting

Women especially, I find, are prone to concerns that intermittent fasting is going to make us feel overly hungry and unproductive, and that it is going to upset our hormones. I've worked hard throughout my career and with all of my patients to dispel these and many other myths associated with fasting. We're going to look at these long-ago disproven notions so that you feel safe and excited about the journey we're on. Here are the myths that I hear the most often.

Myth #1: Intermittent fasting makes you too tired and hungry to be productive

Many women worry that if they fast, they'll be too tired and hungry to focus and be productive. And how can we juggle our work, families, homes, and responsibilities if we can't stay awake or concentrate? Let me reassure you that you'll be more alert and able to focus once you get into the rhythm of fasting. It's one of the reasons that I love this way of eating. Since I started fasting, I've grown my business because I'm more alert and capable than ever. And I don't feel hungry. My patients all say the same thing! Why do we feel less hungry and more alert? Because **we learn to respond to food in a new way.**

After between 4 to 8 hours of not eating, all of us will start to feel hunger pangs. These stomach contractions are triggered by many factors, not all of which are a need for food. You'll know what I mean if you've ever smelled freshly cooked bacon or cinnamon buns and suddenly felt hungry. We have this *unconditioned response* all the time—we pass coffee shops on every street corner, see ads for delicious-looking burgers on our laptops, and breathe in manufactured food smells at the grocery store. And we naturally begin to salivate.

We also have a *conditioned response* to hunger. This response is learned. For example, we feel hungry when we settle in to watch a movie. We eat popcorn because we associate it with a trip to the cinema or a night in front of the TV. We've also conditioned ourselves to be hungry when we get out of bed; at midmorning recess or coffee break; at lunchtime, afternoon recess, or coffee break; suppertime; and in the evening, perhaps when we're sitting in front of our favorite show or just before bed. Much of the time we feel this conditioned response, our bodies are not actually in need of food.

When you fast intermittently, you eat only between certain times on certain days. And to fast successfully, you have to break your conditioned response to food. When you feel hungry because you're sitting on the couch watching a movie, you choose not to eat a bag of chips because you are outside your eating window. You could drink a cup of herbal tea instead. When you feel hungry at midmorning snack, you could take a stretch break instead. As you break these conditioned responses to hunger, and you will, you will feel less hungry. It's liberating to control your eating with such a simple method.

It's worth knowing, too, that fasting is a physiological state in the body, and fasting activates our body's sympathetic nervous system (our fight-or-flight system), which wakes us up and makes us feel energized.

Myth #2: Intermittent fasting causes infertility, interferes with your periods, or upsets your thyroid function

One of the biggest fears women have when considering IF is that fasting will interfere with their hormones, specifically our sex and thyroid hormones. Although female hormones *are* more complicated than male hormones, fasting doesn't affect these hormones in a negative way. In my clinical experience, I've only ever seen fasting affect women in a positive way. Some women do see delays or other irregularities in their menstrual cycle when they first begin fasting. But most women, including many who've struggled to conceive or who have irregular and painful periods, see their menstrual cycle regulate entirely after three months and their symptoms of premenstrual syndrome (PMS) reduced. By regulating our hormones and making our menstrual cycles more predictable, fasting increases fertility. I've worked with women who've been infertile for years who discover after six weeks that they can become pregnant.

Our thyroid hormones are the precursors to our sex hormones, and many women are therefore particularly concerned about fasting negatively affecting their thyroid function. Many women also have thyroid issues unrelated to fertility. The good news is that intermittent fasting improves hypothyroidism and Hashimoto's disease. Both conditions occur when the body makes too little thyroid because the cells become chronically inflamed, and when we fast, we reduce that inflammation, and the cells once again start to take up thyroid hormones efficiently. (If you are taking thyroid medication, consult your endocrinologist before you begin to fast. Many women suddenly experience hyperthyroidism after they start to fast and need to reduce their thyroid medication.)

Myth #3: Intermittent fasting causes your muscles to waste or burn away

Many women worry that if they fast intermittently to lose weight, they will waste or burn away muscle mass. *Wasting* and *burning* both suggest muscle loss: the first because people have the idea that they are not getting enough fuel to maintain muscle integrity, and the second because the assumption is the body somehow uses the muscles for energy. I prefer the term *wasting* because in my clinical experience many people believe muscle wasting happens because the body isn't getting protein when fasting. The body does waste some muscle for protein, but it produces a hormonal cocktail that enables muscle to regrow rapidly when you eat again.

A lot of this thinking about wasting comes from our cultural tendencies, which lead us to overeat. In North America, our government-created food guides tell us to eat six small meals a day plus snacks, and they emphasize grains, cereals, and dairy. Overeating as a lifestyle is built into newer neighborhoods by having a coffee shop on every street corner and a fast-food outlet every few blocks. The result is that most of us are lacking micronutrients because we don't eat enough raw, unprocessed foods, and we're storing a lot of excess fuel energy in our fat cells from eating too much food too often, much of it highly processed and refined. Our bodies want and need to get rid of all that stored fat, which happens when we fast; our muscles don't waste away.

Consider the following analogy. You have 100 pieces of firewood on the porch of a cabin in the woods. You want to make a fire on a cold winter's night. Do you throw the coffee table, which is functional like our muscles, into the fireplace? Or do you use the firewood, which like our body fat has only one purpose as fuel? Why would you chop up a coffee table that serves many uses? Just as you'd burn the more economical firewood as fuel, our bodies use their more economical option: our fat sources. We've evolved to cope with times of food scarcity and food abundance, and this stored fat makes it easy to retrieve fuel when food sources are scarce.

Fasting improves our ability to create lean muscle mass. As we get older, we lose a lot of muscle mass, and muscles are really protective of our joints and organs. Losing muscle mass puts us at risk of losing bone density too. One of the building blocks we need to develop lean mass (muscle and bone mass) is human growth hormone (HGH). And one way to ensure we get enough HGH is to fast. We produce HGH when fasting. In fact, randomized controlled trials show that intermittent fasting retains three times more lean mass than calorie-reduction diets do.[1] So, fasting will help you *gain* muscle strength and bone density.

Another big concern for some women is that fasting will burn muscle. Some fasting naysayers claim (without any evidence) that you lose a quarter pound of muscle for every day of fasting. Considering that I fast at least two days a week and have done so for years, if that were true I shouldn't have enough muscle to type these words. Funny how that hasn't happened. Looking again at those randomized controlled trials, the group eating a calorie-restricted diet lost statistically significant amounts of lean mass, but the group fasting intermittently did not. I believe the fasting group likely lost *less* lean muscle because fasting caused their bodies to pump out HGH and noradrenaline. The fasting group increased lean mass by 2.2 percent whereas the group eating a calorie-restricted diet added only 0.5 percent. In other words, fasting is four times better at preserving lean mass.[2]

Myth #4: Intermittent fasting slows down your metabolism

Many people believe that intermittent fasting slows down our metabolism. This idea is similar to the concern in Myth #1 (that we'll be tired and unproductive), but this myth focuses on the ways that women feel fasting will inhibit specific body processes that will make it impossible to lose weight in the long term.

Fasting activates our sympathetic nervous system, our fight-or-flight response, which produces noradrenaline. This hormone not only helps us to burn body fat and feel energized when we're fasting, but it also preserves our resting metabolic rate (RMR). We'll get into those mechanics in more detail in Chapter 2, but RMR is the energy we expend for breathing, vision, cardiovascular function, and the other basic subconscious systems that keep us alive whether we are asleep or awake.

When we fast, RMR expends more energy even when we relax. However, we don't experience more fatigue because our bodies use our stored fat to give us energy and vitality. A 2016 study shows a clinically significant reduction in RMR in those following a calorie-restricted diet but no reduction in the IF group.[3] In other words, people who are fasting intermittently are using their stored fat sources as fuel, the way our bodies are designed to. Fasting clears out and uses up extra "gas canisters," maintaining our RMR, giving us more energy, and improving our health.

Myth #5: Intermittent fasting causes you to eat more food and less healthy food

Fasting actively burns stored fat to provide your body with all of the calories and energy it needs to function optimally; therefore, appetite is reduced. Also, fasting lowers your primary hunger hormone, ghrelin, and increases your primary satiation hormone, leptin. Most people who are fasting are surprised by how little they want to eat. Their body is fueled by so much of their own fat that they can't physically eat much, even when they break their fast. Is fasting a different experience for women than it is for men? Yes, it is, as we'll see in Chapter 8. Do our end results differ? No, not really. Women just take slightly different routes to get to the same place.

When I finished my first-ever three-day (72-hour) fast, I was so mentally excited to eat that I planned out an amazing break-fast stir-fry. But I was only able to eat a quarter of what I'd prepared because I felt so full! So much body fat was fueling my system that I was left without the urgent need to eat and eat and eat. Because my body was helping me reach an optimal weight for my health, I could relax around food, enjoy my meals, and not overeat. And we see similar results with patients: they eat reasonable, healthy meals when they return to eating.

Junk food can make people who fast feel tired. If, after fasting, you eat foods that fill you up but have no nutritional value—what we call *carbage*—you notice it right away because your system is so clean and efficient. It's like if your car windshield was filthy, you wouldn't notice if a speck of dirt landed on it. But if you washed your windshield and then a speck of dirt or bird poop landed on it, you'd notice immediately. Here's how we answered a question about overeating on our blog.

Does fasting lead to overeating? This was answered in a study published in 2002.[4] Twenty-four healthy subjects underwent a 36-hour fast and then caloric intake was measured. At baseline, subjects ate 2,436 calories per day. After a 36-hour fast, there was an increase in caloric intake to 2,914 calories. So, there was a degree of overeating—almost 20 percent. However, over the two-day period, there was still a net deficit of 1,958 calories. The amount "over" eaten did not nearly compensate for the period of time fasting. The study concluded that a 36-hour fast "did not induce a powerful, unconditioned stimulus to compensate on the subsequent day."

Here's the "spare me the details" bottom line: *no*, fasting does not lead to overeating. No, you will *not* be overwhelmed with hunger.

— DR. JASON FUNG

Myth #6: Intermittent fasting leads to binge eating or eating disorders

A frequent concern I hear from my clients is that fasting will cause them to develop a disordered approach to eating. But because you don't have to count calories or measure foods when you fast, I find their attitude toward food actually becomes more relaxed and healthy. During the times that clients eat, they enjoy their food. When they are fasting, they enjoy how well they feel mentally and physically overall. That's my own story too.

When I was fourteen, I was hospitalized for anorexia. At the time, I felt that my mother was micromanaging me, down to how I tied my shoes and brushed my teeth, and my body image became all important. I wanted to lose a little weight, and I realized the one thing my mother couldn't control was my eating. It began as a revolt against my mother, but my relationship with food became a full-blown eating disorder. Interestingly, once I learned about fasting years later, I became a foodie. I learned I could control my hormonal response and my health; I learned to cook better (setting two kitchens on fire in the process!); and I went from being terrified of food to having a positive relationship with it. I used to have a very limited diet because I was concerned about gaining weight or worsening my metabolic disease. Now I have a set of tools to help me manage my health; I eat a wider range of foods than ever before; and I am able to fast and eat and really enjoy both. I wish that relationship with food for all of you.

THE MYTHS I'VE covered here worry many women as they consider intermittent fasting for the first time, but as I've broken down each one for you, hopefully you feel confident that together we're going to find the IF method that works with your body. We all have hurdles that we need to respect, which means we all need to find our own path to health. Fasting is that solution.

Ava's Story

Ava was thirty-one and desperately wanted to have a baby. She and her husband had been trying for eighteen months to get pregnant. Although her doctor told her she needed to lose weight, every diet Ava tried had failed. They couldn't afford fertility treatment, and so Ava decided to try fasting. When she first came to see me, she was very nervous. She was scared that she wouldn't get enough nutrients, that her metabolic rate would crash and she'd gain weight, and that her menstrual cycles would be disrupted. She was struggling with PCOS, and after we talked about how intermittent fasting might help, she was willing to give it a try.

She soon realized that she had more energy on her fasting days than her eating days. She began to lose fat, which she hadn't been able to do while dieting. But her period, which was usually irregular due to PCOS, became even more irregular. For the first two months, Ava was very afraid that her fertility was being negatively affected. I explained that for some women, it can take three to four months for the hormones in their body to regulate, especially if they have multiple health issues.

Within four months, Ava's menstrual cycles regularized to every twenty-eight days, and her symptoms of PMS started to go away. And her cravings for unhealthy food and her feelings of insecurity began to fade. These results convinced her to keep going with IF. She continued to have fast days and days when she ate healthily, and she lost weight and felt better and better. Within nine months, Ava and her husband conceived naturally! Best of all, Ava's overall health and weight improved through intermittent fasting.

Stories like Ava's can help you to picture how fasting might have a positive impact for you and your own wellness journey. One thing many of my clients have in common is that they've tried various diets before they come to me. And none of these diets have kept their excess weight off, resolved their type 2 diabetes, or improved their fertility. Chances are those diets haven't worked for you either. In the next chapter, you'll learn why.

Chapter 1 Takeaways

- There are several different ways to use intermittent fasting or time-restricted eating, and we each need to find the protocol that best suits our life and body.

- The benefits of intermittent fasting include disease reversal, better health, better hormone regulation, better weight management, and greater personal control of your body, your schedule, and your health.

- The myths around intermittent fasting are pervasive but do not hold up in clinical practice.

- Fasting is a physiological state that activates our body's sympathetic nervous system (fight-or-flight system). When activated, this system triggers hormones that lead to an overall improvement in our wellness.

2

Calorie Confusion
Why Conventional
Dieting Advice Fails

• • • • •

*"Once we understand that obesity is a
hormonal imbalance, we can begin to treat it.
If we believe that excess calories cause obesity, then the
treatment is to reduce calories. But this method has been a
complete failure. However, if too much insulin causes obesity,
then it becomes clear we need to lower insulin levels."*

DR. JASON FUNG

MANY WOMEN COME to me in despair. They've been trying for
years to follow conventional dieting advice but they've not
kept weight off. Often, they initially lost a few pounds on a diet, but
as time went by, they gained it all back, often ending up weighing
more than they did to begin with. Women who diet using conventional dieting advice lose, on average, 10 percent of their starting
weight. This sounds like an okay number, although not incredible, but if you look at that small reduction over a longer time span,
you'll see that most women regain all but 2 pounds within two to
five years of ending their diet.[1]

In this chapter, we'll look at why conventional diets fail us in the long term. We'll go back to basics to see the false assumptions that most dietary advice is based upon and spend some time thinking about how the body really works. But before we do that, let's begin with a word we hear all the time that's at the root of a lot of the confusion: *calorie*.

What Is a Calorie, Really?

We see the word *calorie* on all our nutritional packaging, and many of us associate it with fat or weight gain. But a calorie is simply a measure of energy: one calorie is one unit of energy. Our bodies need energy (measured in calories) to fuel all of our bodily systems, such as our reproductive, respiratory, and cardiovascular functions.

The reason we see calories on our nutritional packaging is that we get our energy (fuel) from food and drinks. Those numbers on our packages tell us how much energy is in a specific portion of that food or drink. The process by which our bodies convert what we eat and drink into energy is called *metabolism*. During this complex process, the calories in our food and drinks are combined with oxygen to release the energy our body needs to function. There's a lot of misinformation about calories, and so it's important to remember that calories are energy. And our bodies need energy.

Conventional dietary advice talks about "calories in" and "calories out." The rest of this chapter uses *Calories In* to refer to the calories we consume in food and drink. *Calories Out* is how calories are used: we "burn" calories as the fuel necessary to move (such as during exercise) and also as the fuel for all of our bodies' systems and functions (such as those associated with our resting metabolic rate).

Many of us have heard that an adult woman needs to consume between 1,600 and 2,400 calories a day to keep her body operating optimally, and many of us have been told that the way to achieve weight loss is to lower the number of calories we consume. Some diets advocate for very low calorie consumption, such as the 1,500-calorie-a-day model (Dr. Ancel Keys's semistarvation diet). The underlying notion is that by reducing our Calories In, we can easily lose weight. However, this idea is not based on fact or current research.

Many of us, however, fundamentally believe that if we reduce Calories In or increase Calories Out, then we will lose weight. We believe that we need to eat less (reduce Calories In) and move more (increase Calories Out)—if only we exercised more, we'd use more calories and lose more weight.

Why the Calorie-Reduction Model Doesn't Work

All current weight-loss diets are founded on the same underlying principle: the number of calories we take in must be less than number of calories we use up. Each dietary trend comes packaged differently: some are soup, shake, and juice diets; others ask you to follow a meal plan or track points. But the underlying principle is the same caloric equation. We may try this meal plan or that juice diet, but the results are always the same. We lose some weight and then regain it all. We try a new diet. Same results. We try another diet. No change. One definition of insanity is doing the same thing repeatedly and expecting different results. Conventional weight-loss diets are nothing short of insanity.

In scientific circles, this approach is known as *caloric reduction as a primary strategy* or simply the *calorie-reduction model*. And reducing calories is done in one of two ways: either by decreasing how many calories we consume in food and drink or by increasing how many calories we burn off by moving our bodies. Although each diet may have its particular set of rules, at the core they are all structured like this:

Calories In < Calories Out

Or maybe you've heard or seen it as:

Eat Less, Move More

Whether you get a fast-food burger from McDonald's, Burger King, or Wendy's, a burger is a burger. Similarly, it doesn't matter if your diet advises shakes, soups, fish, or various other options, they all have the same principle at heart. Every weight-loss diet you've tried is founded on the Calories In < Calories Out philosophy—and this principle is *not working*. It's built on several assumptions that have been around for a long time, all of which are false.

The three false assumptions I hear most often are:

1 Calories In and Calories Out are independent.

2 We have conscious control of Calories In.

3 We have conscious control of Calories Out.

We'll look at each of these false assumptions, and then we'll start asking some questions together: this is the approach I take with my clients in person, and it's transformative as they realize they're not the ones doing anything wrong! I know many women feel like they have failed and are endlessly frustrated by their own bodies because they don't lose weight no matter the diet they follow. What I want you to get out of this chapter is that conventional dietary advice *itself* is the failure, not you or any of the women who've found it impossible to manage their weight.

The body tends toward homeostasis

The first false assumption is that Calories In and Calories Out are independent. To understand weight gain and weight loss, we need to understand what happens *between* calories coming in and calories going out. They are linked hormonally and through complex body systems. The body determines what it uses (Calories In) and what it doesn't (Calories Out), and the notion that we have conscious control over this balance causes a lot of harm to women as they try to lose weight. (In fact, the second and third false assumptions I most often hear are both corollaries of this primary false assumption.)

The truth is that Calories In and Calories Out are *not* independent because our bodies have a tendency toward balance, or equilibrium, in all systems. This tendency is called *homeostasis*. When fewer calories come into the body, the body slows down so it uses fewer of them. The false assumption that Calories In are independent of Calories Out ignores the importance of homeostasis and the body's tendency to balance. Let's explore this idea further.

In conventional dieting advice, the energy balance equation is usually stated as Body Fat = Calories In – Calories Out. This equation is almost always *misinterpreted* to mean that if we simply eat fewer calories or exercise more, we'll lose body fat. And this thinking has informed dieting advice for the past fifty years. We've been told to restrict calories by eating less dietary fat—foods like butter, cheese, nuts, eggs, and meat that are calorie dense. We've also been told to reduce the number of calories we consume by controlling our portion size—putting less on our plate or eating small amounts many times a day, instead of larger meals. But remember, there are *three* variables to consider: Body Fat, Calories In, and Calories Out.

We've been led to believe that our bodies always need the same number of calories to keep running normally. By that thinking, if you change one variable, say, Calories In, then either Body Fat or Calories Out may change to keep the equation stable. This idea assumes that body fat is simply an unregulated receptacle for excess calories. But it's not. And this is because of our resting metabolic rate (RMR).

The RMR is the number of calories that the body burns as it performs the functions it needs to stay alive. RMR is also often called the basal metabolic rate (BMR). Think of this rate as the number of calories your body would need if you just stayed in bed all day long! Even to get through a day when we're not moving at all, calories are essential fuel for basic bodily functions. These basic functions—such as keeping our heart pumping, our brain thinking, our lungs breathing, and our liver detoxifying—burn calories at a certain rate. That rate varies from person to person, and RMR changes throughout our lives too.

The bottom line is that the body can adjust its resting metabolic rate. What this means is that when you eat fewer calories, your body slows down its RMR: it uses fewer calories. As a result, long term, you don't lose weight. We'll dive into how the body regulates RMR later in the book, particularly in the later chapters about hormones, but for now it's important to understand that all human body systems are tightly regulated. We are highly complex animals with many interdependent organ systems, and this tight regulation is essential for us to survive. This tight regulation applies to every part of human physiology. And what it means is that body fat is not a landfill of excess calories but part of a complex system, balanced by our hormones and our RMR.

Hormones regulate how the body stores energy

The second false assumption is that we have conscious control of Calories In. The calorie-reduction model assumes a causal relationship between eating too much and obesity. That is, eating too many calories causes obesity, and therefore the solution is to eat less (fewer calories). The dieting world has many options for eating less: cut out sugar, fast food, processed foods, and so on. All of these diets assume that eating too much is the primary cause of obesity. Following this flawed logic, we might ask, "Why is somebody eating too many calories?" The answer would be "It's a personal choice."

We can test the hypothesis that we have conscious control of Calories In by adjusting how many calories are eaten. What happens when you restrict calories? The standard point of view predicts that eating fewer calories has no impact on the number of Calories Out or on your resting metabolic rate (RMR). That if you eat less, then you lose weight. We've all heard this sort of advice: eat 500 fewer calories per day and lose 1 pound of body fat per week. But as we know, often from personal experience, that's not what happens. And study after study, as we'll see in a minute, confirms it.

Pretend for a moment that calories are money you spend in an energy budget for the body. Let's say your household income is reduced by 30 percent. In the short term, you may find that you're overspending because you're not used to your budget cut. You may get into some debt. But a month or two down the road, you start to cut your expenses. Maybe you purchase a Netflix subscription instead of going to the movies or take public transit instead of using your car. Over time, you stop overspending and adjust to your new budget.

That's what happens in calorie-restriction diets. In the short term, you continue to overspend and so you lose some weight. But in the long term, your body cuts costs and starts to use less energy. Your body learns to accommodate: it cuts costs from your cognitive function, your reproductive system, and other systems in the body. As a result, you feel awful. Your brain gets foggy. You're hungry all the time. Most people can't function with this unsustainable model, and so they return to their old way of eating. Because they have cut energy use across the board, they come across the biggest problem with calorie restriction: when they return to eating the way they did *before* the calorie-restriction diet, they start to gain weight.

Calorie-restriction diets lower our metabolic rate; the body can no longer use up its typical calorie intake *because* of the diet. The cycle of some weight loss and overall weight gain continues. That's when you try a new diet with a different name. But the soup or smoothie or point-counting diet is the same diet with different packaging. And none of them work. The calorie-reduction model ignores the fact that fat stores are *hormonally* regulated, as we'll see in Chapter 3. None of these calorie-restriction diets address the root cause of obesity, which is hormone related and goes by the name *insulin resistance*.

Hormones regulate how the body uses energy

The third false assumption is that we have conscious control of Calories Out. Just as the calorie-reduction model assumes a causal relationship between eating too much and obesity, it also assumes a causal relationship between obesity and too little exercise. That is, not using enough calories causes obesity, and therefore the solution is to move more. The fitness world has many options for exercising more, like high-intensity interval training (HIIT), body-sculpting classes, and so on, but none of these methods of increasing Calories Out deals with the root cause of obesity. If you've been made to feel lazy or less than because you can't shift your weight with exercise, you're not alone. But exercise is not the key to weight loss.

Hormones regulate how our body uses energy, and you can exercise as much as you like but see no impact on your weight (a situation many of you will recognize) because the number of calories that "go out" are not relevant to your weight management.

Real-Life Evidence That the Calorie-Reduction Model Doesn't Work

The Biggest Loser is a long-running American TV reality show that pits obese contestants against one another in a bid to lose the most weight. Currently, the *Biggest Loser* diet is ranked as the twentieth most popular diet, and I'd like to explore the impact it has had upon our collective cultural understanding of food and weight loss. The weight-loss regimen is a calorie-restricted diet calculated to be approximately 70 percent of the contestants' energy requirements, typically 1,200 to 1,500 calories per day, plus an intensive exercise regimen typically far in excess of two hours daily. As this classic eat less, move more approach is endorsed by all the nutritional authorities, *The Biggest Loser* diet scored third on *USA Today*'s 2015 ranking of best weight-loss diets. The average weight lost per contestant that season was 127 pounds over six months, which shows that this method absolutely does work in the *short term*. But does it work long term? Season 2's contestant Suzanne Mendonca said it best when she explained that there is never a reunion show because "We're all fat again."[2]

On the *Biggest Loser* diet, the resting metabolic rate (RMR) drops like a piano from a twenty-story building. Over six months in 2015, contestants' RMR dropped by an average of 789 calories. Simply stated, they burned 789 fewer calories per day, every day. As metabolism drops, weight loss plateaus. The body shuts down its basic functions to match the lowered caloric intake. Once expenditure drops below intake, weight is regained—this happens for contestants after the cameras stop rolling and the show is done. Goodbye reunion show. Even after six years, the metabolic rate does not recover. This result is completely predictable. Everyone regains weight despite following a calorie-restricted diet, even as your friends and family silently accuse you of cheating on your diet.

Metabolic slowdown has been scientifically proven for over fifty years. Eat less, move more works only in the short term, before resting metabolism falls in response. Daily calorie restriction fails because it puts you into metabolic slowdown, or starvation mode. It's a guarantee. What you need to know is this: the secret to long-term weight loss is to *maintain your resting metabolism*. What I'll share with you about fasting will help you keep your RMR stable, but first let's look at what science shows us about why conventional diets don't work.

Scientific Evidence That the Calorie-Reduction Model Doesn't Work

In the 1950s, Dr. Ancel Keys's famous Minnesota starvation experiment placed volunteers on a "semistarvation" diet of 1,500 calories per day, which was 30 percent fewer calories than their previous diet.[3] In response, their resting metabolic rate dropped about 30 percent. They felt cold, tired, and hungry. When they resumed their typical diet, all their weight came right back. Since then, many other researchers have carried out randomized controlled trials to test various theories about weight loss.

The Women's Health Initiative Study

Published in 2006, the Women's Health Initiative (WHI) dietary modification trial was an expensive and ambitious National Institutes of Health study that followed close to 50,000 postmenopausal women in the United States for an average of 7.5 years with start dates between 1993 and 1998.[4] Postmenopausal women were chosen because menstruation introduces too much variability; PCOS or sex hormone variables interfere with results, so such research is often, if not exclusively, conducted with postmenopausal women. The results are still useful for all women to show the impacts of Calories In and Calories Out on weight and metabolic health.

The women in this study either ate their usual diet (control group) or a calorie-restricted, low-fat diet in line with guidelines endorsed and accepted by virtually all medical professionals (study group). The study group ate less and exercised more. The study group received education sessions, group activities, interviews, and personalized feedback to reduce dietary fat to 20 percent of daily calories, increase vegetables and fruit to five servings a day, and increase grains to six servings a day. The control group, by contrast, got a copy of *Dietary Guidelines for Americans*, a booklet that provides general information about healthy eating and special considerations for different populations.

Consistent with the nutritional recommendations of the time, total caloric intake for the study group was lowered from 1,788 to 1,446 calories a day, a reduction of 361.4 calories per day for over seven years. Fat as a percentage of calories was reduced from 38.8 percent at the start of the study to 29.8 percent in later years.

Carbohydrates were increased from 44.5 to 52.7 percent since eating whole grains was encouraged. This group could have expected to lose more than 30 pounds per year in theory. In reality? After 7.5 years, this group weighed about 0.9 pounds less than their starting weight.

Although we haven't yet looked at body fat compared to body weight, you'll see in later chapters how significant body fat is compared to body weight. Body weight is the combination of body fat, muscle, bone, water mass, and other things. You can weigh 97 pounds and still be morbidly obese if you have a lot of body fat.

But back to this study. Despite a slightly lower weight overall, the women following this eat less, move more diet had a larger waist size, suggesting that they carried more of the dangerous fat that accumulates around the midsection. This visceral fat is associated with several serious health issues that affect women, like cardiovascular disease.

The second pillar of this Women's Health Initiative study was an increase in exercise. The women in the study group increased their daily physical activity from 10 METs/week to 11.4 METs/week. A MET is a metabolic equivalent, which measures physical activity or the rate of energy expended over time. The women in the study group increased their level of physical activity by 14 percent over those 7.5 years while following the calorie-restricted, lower-fat diet.

At the beginning of the study, the average weight was 169 pounds (76.8 kg) with an average body mass index (BMI) of 29.1. This index, which measures body fat based on height and weight, is used to classify people as underweight, normal weight, overweight, or obese. So, 29.1 put the women in the overweight category, bordering on obese. What happened over the seven years?

The eat less, move more group started out well with an average of nearly 4.5 pounds (more than 2 kg) of weight loss over the first year. By the second year, they began to regain the weight, and by the end of the study, there was no significant difference between the two groups. Weight loss over 7.5 years was not on average even one single pound. One possible explanation is that the women lost fat and gained muscle and so their weight remained stable. If so, they would have a reduced waist-hip ratio (WHR), since body fat is typically carried around the waist. Unfortunately, the average waist size increased from 35 to 35.5 inches (89.0 to 90.1 cm), and the average WHR increased from 0.82 to 0.83. Not only did these women not lose weight, they were actually fatter than before.

Many people say, "I don't understand. I eat less. I exercise more. But I can't seem to lose any weight." I know. I believe them. Because this advice has been proven to fail.

A separate paper examined the exercise portion of the Women's Health Initiative in more detail. Researchers followed 39,876 women from 1992 to 2004, dividing them into three groups representing high, medium, and low levels of weekly exercise.[5]

The group that exercised the least (<7.5 MET hours per week) did less than about 150 minutes per week, an average of 20 minutes per day. The group that did the most exercise (>21 MET hours per week) did more than an hour a day. At baseline, the women who exercised the most were the lightest, and the ones who exercised the least were the heaviest. So far, so good. But what happened over the next ten years? You might expect that those who continued to exercise would continue to increase their weight-loss benefits. Surprisingly, that's not what the research showed.

If you exercise for one hour every single day for three years, you would expect to weigh an extra quarter pound. That's more than if you did nothing at all. As Eric Ravussin, a diabetes and metabolism researcher at Louisiana State University explained in *Time* magazine, "In general, for weight loss, exercise is pretty useless."[6]

The underwhelming results we see in the WHI study are confirmed in virtually every other randomized controlled trial study that has been done since.

The Diabetes Prevention Program and the Look AHEAD Study

The Diabetes Prevention Program (DPP) was a trial that ran from 1996 to 2001. The program randomly sorted people into one of three groups: one that followed a low-calorie, low-fat diet and did 150 minutes of exercise a week; a group that took 850 milligrams of metformin (a diabetes medication) twice a day; and a placebo group. The DPP outcome study has continued to follow most of the original participants since 2002. Did the eat less diet strategy work for the lifestyle-change group? Hardly. After ten years, there was virtually no weight difference between the people who ate their usual diet and the group that deliberately restricted their calories.[7]

The National Institutes of Health sponsored an even more ambitious effort in 2001. The Look AHEAD (Action for Health in Diabetes) randomized controlled trial studied 5,145 overweight men and women with type 2 diabetes, testing whether an intensive low-calorie diet could reduce heart attacks and strokes.[8] Participants would eat either their usual meals (support and education group) or a diet reduced to between 1,200 and 1,800 calories per day (lifestyle intervention group), combined with increased exercise. The participants following the calorie-restricted diet were able to maintain about a 7-pound weight loss after ten years, compared to those eating their usual diet.

This result sounds pretty good, but it's not quite true if you look a little more closely. If patients in the intervention group were not losing enough weight, the protocol called for their diet to be tightened to as little as 1,000 calories per day. If that dietary restriction didn't maintain their weight loss, they could be given weight-loss drugs. In other words, these results are not a fair comparison of no intervention against the effects of a low-calorie diet alone.

The primary purpose of the study was to show that weight loss could reduce heart attacks and strokes. However, the trial was abandoned after 9.6 years of follow-up because of medical futility. That is, there was virtually no chance that this intervention would be successful, and so the researchers decided there was no point in wasting more time and money on it.

The HEALTHY Study

In 2010, the HEALTHY Study Group published a paper entitled "A School-Based Intervention for Diabetes Risk Reduction" in the prestigious *New England Journal of Medicine*.[9] An increasing number of school-age children are overweight or obese, which puts them at higher risk for type 2 diabetes. The purpose of the study was to evaluate the effects of a three-year multicomponent intervention delivered through schools. A total of 4,603 students in Grades 6 to 8 from forty-two schools took part. Half the students were simply assessed at regular intervals; the other half (the intervention group) were encouraged to:

- lower the average fat content of their food

- eat at least two servings of fruit and vegetables per day

- eat at least two servings of grain-based food and/or legumes per day

- increase their time doing moderate to vigorous physical activity

While the study involved students, in my clinical experience, the results apply to everyone: adults and youth. And it is the same advice we've heard over and over. Did students lose more weight using this approach? Did it work? No, the intervention group saw no measurable benefit compared to the group doing nothing special.

One Last Time: Calories Are Not the Culprit

To sum up, here's what the scientific evidence says about the eat less, move more strategy of weight loss: low-calorie diets combined with increased exercise do *not* result in long-term weight loss. If you combine a low-calorie diet with weight-loss drugs, you can cause mild weight loss (about 3 percent of body weight). However, this strategy does not make you healthier in any measurable way. So, the basic dietary advice that's been given to billions of people all over the world for the last fifty years results in virtually no long-term weight loss and zero impact on health. It's no wonder we have an epidemic of obesity and type 2 diabetes in our culture. Consider the following statistics:

- 52 percent of American adults have at least one chronic illness.[10]

- 70 percent of Americans are overweight or obese.[11]

- On an average diet, people gain back 80 percent of weight lost within five years.[12]

- The average person will try 126 diets in their lifetime.[13]

All of us have been set up to fail. To repeat, because it goes so against everything you've been told: the reason that the dietary advice we've all heard so many times doesn't work is because the secret of weight loss doesn't lie with calorie counting; it has to do with our hormones. We do not have conscious control of either Calories In or Calories Out because our body naturally wants to reach equilibrium (homeostasis). When Calories In goes down, Calories Out also decreases to compensate. And when Calories In goes up, Calories Out also increases to maintain balance. The result is no weight loss. What regulates this homeostasis in the body? Hormones. The sooner we accept that hormones regulate our metabolism and food storage, the sooner we can stop following faulty advice. And the sooner we can stop blaming ourselves for not getting the results we're "supposed" to.

Gisele's Story

Gisele was struggling with her weight. She was in her late forties and had been recently berated by her doctor for not losing weight. She told me how after that experience, she stood in her office, sharing this experience with her colleague. While she was sharing, she ate cookie after cookie. "Should you even be eating those cookies?" her colleague asked.

"These are plant based," Gisele replied, "and they're low fat. It's better I eat this than nothing at all." The cookies she was eating to soothe herself were *on her diet plan*, and they were the right number of points. She was allowed to eat them, and eating them was helping her feel better about the unpleasant conversation with the doctor, which had made her feel so inadequate. What Gisele had never been told was *why* her diet was never going to work and that it wasn't her fault that the diet was failing. Her conversation with her colleague, as she relayed it to me, made her feel even worse and made her want to eat even more to numb her feelings of failure and inadequacy. My heart broke for all the years she'd been made to feel less than and at fault. I knew she was doing everything she'd been told, and I knew why that advice was failing her. Hopefully what you've learned in this chapter helps you see why too.

With my help, Gisele began fasting three times a week on a 42-hour protocol. She cut out snacking and learned why low-fat foods weren't helping her. She changed her mindset to understand that healthy fats were good for her, and now she is maintaining a 60-pound weight loss. She feels fit and healthy and has a great relationship with food (if not with her rude colleague!).

In the next chapter, we'll begin to explore what regulates how much body fat we carry and look at the root cause of obesity and poor metabolic health. Then you'll see how intermittent fasting is different from every other diet you've ever tried.

Chapter 2 Takeaways

- Every diet you've tried is based on the same principles. They're all the same diet with different names, just like toilet paper from different companies is still toilet paper. And none of them will help you to lose weight.

- The commonly accepted dietary advice is based on three false assumptions. We assume that the calories that go into our body and the calories that go out are independent. And that we have conscious control over both. We therefore believe that we can control our body fat if we control our calories by eating less and exercising more. These beliefs are not true.

- Most people regain any weight they lose on a diet not because they have failed but because their body's resting metabolic rate slows down to compensate for fewer calories.

- Exercising more is not a proven strategy for effective weight loss.

- Calorie-restriction diets ignore the biological principle of homeostasis, which is the body's ability to adapt to changing environments. These diets do not address the root cause of obesity.

- It's not your fault that none of the diets you've tried in the past has worked. The scientific evidence does not support the calorie-reduction method.

3

The Role of Insulin Resistance in Obesity and Poor Metabolic Health

. . . . .

"The healthy snack is one of the greatest weight-loss deceptions. The myth that 'grazing is healthy' has attained legendary status. If we were meant to graze, we would be cows. Grazing is the direct opposite of virtually all food traditions. Even as recently as the 1960s, most people still ate just three meals per day. Constant stimulation of insulin eventually leads to insulin resistance."

DR. JASON FUNG

THE REASON THAT intermittent fasting helps us to lose and maintain weight; reverse type 2 diabetes, PCOS, and nonalcoholic fatty liver disease; and lower cholesterol and blood pressure is that it addresses the root cause of the problems. Conventional diets are concerned with calories. But obesity and poor metabolic health are caused by insulin resistance. And insulin is a hormone, so the key to better health is to balance our hormones.

All systems in the body are tightly regulated by specific hormones. Several key hormones regulate metabolism—the process by which the body converts food and drink into fuel. Ghrelin, also known as the hunger hormone, causes hunger. And peptide YY3–36 causes us to feel satisfied and stop eating. But insulin is by far the most important hormone when it comes to metabolism because it regulates energy storage. We can't decide in our heads to feel hungry or full. And we can't decide whether to store energy as fat or use it for fuel. That's insulin's job. Understanding what insulin resistance is and its impact upon health is fundamental to how I help clients transform their relationship with food. In this chapter, I share what I've learned to set you up for your fasting journey.

What Is Insulin?

Insulin is a hormone naturally produced in the body by the pancreas. Many people associate insulin with diabetes because we know someone with the disease, or we have it ourselves. People with type 1 diabetes take insulin because their own pancreas produces little or no insulin naturally. Without that insulin, their bodies would not be able to store or burn energy, and they would die. People with type 2 diabetes produce too much insulin, and their bodies are constantly receiving the message to store more energy. Why does this happen?

When we eat, our stomach and intestines break food down into its component parts: dietary fat, protein, and carbohydrates (macronutrients) as well as vitamins and minerals (micronutrients). The digestive system handles each macronutrient differently. Dietary fat breaks down into fatty acids; protein breaks down into amino acids; and carbohydrates become sugars, including glucose. Insulin helps the body use this glucose, which is floating around in the blood, by getting it inside cells where it provides energy. Glucose will keep floating around in the blood unless it has insulin to help.

If we ask *how* insulin lowers our blood glucose levels, we start to discover the complexities of this hormone. Insulin lowers our blood glucose levels by binding to the insulin receptor on a cell. It's like a key that fits snugly into a lock. When insulin opens up the lock on the cell, glucose can get in to provide the energy the cell needs. Glucose leaves the blood and enters the cell. This is how insulin lowers our blood glucose levels.

But cells only need so much energy—and some don't need energy in that moment. Let's say you're sitting down, watching a movie, *after* dinner. Perhaps you grab yourself a bag of popcorn because you have the conditioned response to snack. Your cells don't need any more energy at that time, and so your body has to decide what to do with the extra energy that you're consuming. Insulin's job is to figure out how to store the excess energy.

The body can store excess food energy in two ways, as:

1 glycogen in the liver or

2 body fat

When food enters the body, insulin signals to the liver that nutrients are on their way. Our intestines deliver amino acids and glucose directly to the liver. Whatever energy the liver can't use right away, it strings together into long chains to form the molecule glycogen. Our glycogen reserves are little energy packs for when the body needs a quick hit of fuel. They're kept in our muscles and in our liver. The glycogen packs stored in the liver can easily be converted to and from glucose to quickly supply energy to different parts of the body. The glycogen packs stored in muscles can only be used by the muscles.

When we eat and drink, insulin decides what to do with any extra fuel we consume. Insulin will first assess glycogen reserves. And here there's a catch. Our body has limited capacity to store glycogen in our muscles and liver (because they have other functions).

The excess fuel, once the glycogen stores are full, gets redirected into our fat cells. This happens through a complex metabolic pathway called de novo lipogenesis. Essentially, the body sends extra glucose or glycogen to fat cells for long-term storage.

Think of insulin as a traffic controller for the energy (glucose) that comes in as food.

Insulin directs:

1 energy to cells

2 energy to glycogen packs

When there's no more needed energy:

3 the excess is directed to stuff our fat cells

Now that we know more about how insulin works in the body, we'll dive more deeply into the way it impacts our fat cells and our weight.

The Link Between Insulin and Obesity

We all have fat cells. When we lose weight, we don't lose the fat cells; we just lose their fullness. We empty out the excess energy inside them. Sometimes our fat cells are empty and we weigh less. Sometimes they're full and we weigh more. Ultimately, insulin is responsible for the change because its job is to direct the storage of excess food energy in the body.

Interestingly, doctors can make *anyone* gain weight by giving them insulin. The average type 2 diabetic on insulin gains about 5 to 10 pounds around their belly within one month of starting their injections. Even without injections, we can lead our body to overproduce insulin. One way is through *high stress and poor sleep*, which we'll explore in Chapter 5. We can also exacerbate the problem through *what we eat*. A standard American diet (SAD), which emphasizes grains and starches, encourages insulin production. Remember, carbohydrates break down into glucose. We can also lead our body to overproduce insulin through *how often we eat*. The more often we snack and graze, the more we stimulate insulin production.

Together, these three factors lead the body to produce too much insulin. Hyperinsulinemia means the amount of insulin in the blood is higher than what's considered normal. Ultimately, hyperinsulinemia leads to insulin resistance. This resistance is the root cause of obesity.

How we develop insulin resistance

When we live with chronic stress or snack and graze all the time, especially when those foods are high in sugar or refined carbohydrates, we increase insulin secretion in the body. That constant secretion, in turn, overstimulates our body's insulin production. After a while, the insulin receptors on our cells become less receptive, and it takes more insulin to open the gates to the cells. At some point, the receptors stop working with our own insulin. No one really understands why from a biochemical perspective, although we know that it happens. When it does, it's called insulin resistance (IR). Our insulin and our receptors aren't compatible anymore, and we develop type 2 diabetes or obesity.

Insulin resistance leads to an accumulation of even more insulin in the blood. Even when cells need energy, they don't get it because insulin can't engage the insulin receptor and so glucose isn't allowed into the cell. This abnormal glucose metabolism causes fatigue—this is why people who are overweight or have type 2 diabetes always feel so tired. We see high glucose levels in these people; glucose builds up in the blood because it can't get into the cells. Researchers believe this condition is caused by chronic exposure to insulin, which can lead to toxic levels of insulin in the body.

Here's an analogy. My favorite singer is Adele. Back when her hit single "Hello" came out, I loved it. Everyone loved it. It won a billion awards—and it was on the radio all the time. One day as I was driving home from work, "Hello" was playing on eight of the twelve preset radio stations in my car. I realized I was sick of Adele and just wanted to shout "Goodbye!" when she sang "Hello." I'd developed Adele resistance due to overexposure. Several months later, after radio stations moved on to play other music, I liked the song again. We can all develop resistance from overexposure.

So, the more insulin you have in your blood, the more sugar you have in your blood, which ultimately leads to type 2 diabetes. Typically, doctors treat the symptom of type 2 diabetes by giving the patient insulin, but the root cause is usually that insulin and the body's insulin receptors aren't working together anymore. And so we often give diabetics more and more insulin. Too much insulin also stimulates growth, which can lead to PCOS (growths on the ovaries) and obesity (more fuel being stored for later).

You don't have to have type 2 diabetes to be insulin resistant. In fact, many of us are on our way to type 2 diabetes without even knowing it. When we eat six small meals a day and snack, as many of our current food guidelines and diet plans suggest, we cause insulin to be secreted all day long. Imagine the phone started ringing every time you ate and your body started to secrete insulin. If the phone is ringing every hour, you're quickly going to get tired of the noise and develop resistance too.

In addition to the insulin that's secreted when you are stressed or when you eat, insulin resistance *itself* causes the body to secrete insulin! Most people who seek out my program have been following a low-carb or a ketogenic diet for some time, and their insulin levels are already in the prediabetic range. But they can't lose those last few pounds of excess weight. Very often, the problem is that they went from eating foods that caused the body to secrete high levels of insulin to a diet that has them eating constantly. Despite changing *what* they eat (choosing more healthful options), they have not changed *when* they eat—and they are still constantly producing insulin. The volume and frequency of that insulin secretion leads to insulin resistance. If you often eat foods that cause a lot of insulin secretion, you can perpetuate this cycle even if you aren't insulin resistant.

The damage of constantly fueling

In modern life, food has become our best friend. We eat to celebrate, to comfort ourselves, to relieve boredom. We're constantly fueling!

We overwhelm our bodies with insulin in two ways. First, we eat too much all at once, which produces great *surges* of insulin. Think of eating a very heavy meal as like 100 people knocking on your front door all at the same time. Eating a big plate of something high in carbohydrates, like pasta, produces a lot of insulin that overwhelms the body. Second, we eat all the time, which produces a *constant stimulus* of insulin. One person knocking on your door every hour of the day would also become overwhelming by the end of the day. In the same way, a steady secretion of insulin overwhelms us.

Consider a typical day for many people:

Wake up
Eat breakfast
Get to work
Eat a snack on a coffee break
Eat lunch
Eat an afternoon snack
Go for a walk or to the gym
Eat a snack before dinner
Eat dinner
Eat a snack while watching TV (or meet a friend for a drink and snack)
Eat a snack before bed
Go to bed

Even if you are only snacking on nuts, seeds, cheese, and olives, and choosing healthy fats at mealtimes, you are still having a nonstop insulin response throughout the day. It's not that you can't eat those foods, you just need to eat them with a meal to minimize the *frequency* of insulin secretion. We'll look carefully at different types of food and their impacts in the next chapter, but note that even if you're eating healthily, the damage of constantly fueling is immense.

If you are eating frequently, you cannot heal your body. Imagine that the government says you must fill your vehicle's gas tank every day. They insist that you fill 16 gallons *daily*. But you only drive 6 miles per day. You'd need to buy gas canisters to put the extra fuel in. As you fill up one canister, you'll need another and another and another. Eventually your car, backyard, garage, and whole house would be full—and you're living in a hazard zone with gas canisters everywhere! When we eat constantly, that's what we do: we keep storing fat in our fat cells until we cause chronic illnesses, such as obesity and metabolic syndrome.

The Link Between Insulin and Metabolic Syndrome (MetS)

Metabolic syndrome (MetS) describes a group of symptoms that puts us at high risk for developing cardiovascular disease, type 2 diabetes, nonalcoholic fatty liver disease (NAFLD), polycystic ovary syndrome (PCOS), and metabolic-related cancers, such as breast cancer (if it is not genetic)[1] or colon cancer. The symptoms of MetS are:

- high blood sugar
- large waist circumference
- high triglycerides

- low HDL (high-density lipoprotein or "good") cholesterol

- high blood pressure

Insulin resistance is the root cause of MetS. But just as everyone who is exposed to coronavirus doesn't experience all COVID-19 symptoms, everyone who has insulin resistance won't get all of its associated symptoms. And when we manage our insulin resistance, we manage our symptoms and treat our diseases.

We'll discuss PCOS and some female cancers in Chapter 7, but I want to take a moment to consider type 2 diabetes. The most common medical intervention for type 2 diabetes is to treat it with insulin. But if insulin resistance is the cause of type 2 diabetes, why do we do this?

Type 2 diabetes

The current standard of care for type 2 diabetes treats the high blood glucose (blood sugar) levels. Insulin medications lower the blood sugar to "normal" levels, but remember that high blood sugar is the symptom, not the cause. These medications move the sugar from the blood and store it *elsewhere* in the body, causing obesity, inflammation, and disease. It's like taking all of the garbage from your kitchen and putting it in your basement. Yes, your kitchen looks cleaner, but your house is still just as messy. Because the medications lower blood glucose levels and patients aren't being seen daily, they're told to eat several times a day and to consume high-sugar foods to "stabilize blood sugar levels." In other words, they're told to eat sugar so the medications don't make their sugar levels go too low. This advice makes no sense at all.

A ninety-year-old man at my grandmother's nursing home understood this. He couldn't work out why if his morning blood sugar reading was 140 mg/dL, he needed to eat sugar to bring that reading up and then take his medication to bring it back down to the same 140 mg/dL level. He asked why he couldn't just fast to burn off the sugar. He was right. The nurse practitioner wouldn't answer him, so I pushed for an answer. She threw me out. There is a lot of resistance to the idea of fasting as a solution for type 2 diabetes, but the more information you have, and the more support you have from a health professional who understands fasting, the easier it is to make choices around fasting that best suit your health journey.

Insulin is absolutely necessary for type 1 diabetics because their body doesn't produce it, but type 2 diabetes is a disease of too much insulin caused by lifestyle and dietary factors. Insulin relieves the symptoms of type 2 diabetes, but it *does not treat the root cause*. So, how do we prevent and reverse insulin resistance and the diseases that follow from it?

Insulin Sensitivity, Intermittent Fasting, and Breaking the Cycle of Insulin Resistance

The opposite of insulin resistance is insulin sensitivity. The receptors on our cells work with our own insulin, and the cells get the energy that they need. *We want our cells to be insulin sensitive.*

Here is the key to understanding why intermittent fasting helps address the root cause of obesity, insulin resistance. Just like when I took a break from listening to Adele, when we fast intermittently, we suppress insulin for long periods of time and give the body a break. And then when we break our fast and reexpose the body to insulin, our cells become more insulin sensitive. Insulin works again the way it's supposed to in our bodies, just like when I went back to listening to Adele and loved the song "Hello" anew!

So, how do we lower insulin in the body? My answer for thousands of clients is that to lower insulin surges in the body, we lower stress and get more sleep (as we explore in Chapter 5), eat fewer high-glucose foods (Chapter 4), and eat less often. And that's where intermittent fasting comes in. Unlike calorie restriction, a low carbohydrate, high healthy fat diet combined with intermittent fasting keeps insulin levels in balance. Fasting suppresses insulin production for an extended period of time, breaking the cycle of insulin resistance. For many of my clients, this changes their lives!

Marge's Story

Marge was seventy-two when she first came to see me at the Toronto clinic. She was struggling to manage her weight and type 2 diabetes. Every time she saw her doctor, he told her she needed to take ten more units of insulin. And every time, she gained 10 pounds. During the course of her illness and treatment, she'd gained 110 pounds on the 110 units of insulin she was taking. Marge had been diabetic for thirty-four years and been on insulin for the last seven. She felt awful and told me that she didn't want to live anymore.

I looked over her charts. *Every* time she added more insulin, she gained exactly the same number of pounds. We needed to break the cycle, and so I suggested an extended fast. Dr. Jason Fung was the medical doctor who monitored her as she fasted for a total of seven days to start. Marge was feeling so good that we decided to continue her fast for another two weeks. While that prolonged fast worked well for Marge, I don't want any of you leaping into that type of fast—especially without medical supervision—and crashing and burning. Keep reading and go slowly!

Marge was the first person I'd asked to fast, and so I fasted along with her. After seven days, her insulin was reduced—by *50 percent*! She continued to fast, and by the end of twenty-one days, she was off all her insulin and her blood glucose levels were normal. After six months, she had a totally normal hemoglobin A1C test, an average of blood glucose levels over three months, which is our measure for diabetes. Within a year, she'd lost 110 pounds. More importantly, she'd regained her joy in life and was thriving.

Marge would often come to the IDM clinic and talk to the other doctors working there about her experience with fasting. She would come to grand rounds and journal club to share her story with our colleagues. They were at first unsure about our fasting approach, but they soon understood the incredible benefits of fasting.

Having seen Marge's health improve with fasting, her husband started to fast as well, which helped him lose weight. He was able to come off his diabetic medication and reverse his diabetes too. Marge and her husband began to enjoy their renewed energy and zest for life together.

In this chapter, we've looked at the harm caused by *when we eat* (that is, constant fueling). This is the first of three factors that lead the body to overproduce insulin, which leads to insulin resistance, obesity, and the metabolic diseases that flow from it. Next, we'll explore the second of the three factors: the types of food we consume in a standard American diet, or *what we eat*, and how our food choices impact our bodies.

Chapter 3 Takeaways

- Insulin is a hormone produced by the pancreas that directs how the body uses food energy as fuel.

- Our dietary habits lead to insulin resistance in two main ways: eating the standard American diet (SAD) produces large surges of insulin, and eating all the time (snacking and grazing) creates a constant stimulus of insulin.

- Insulin resistance is the root cause of obesity. It causes a whole host of symptoms known as metabolic syndrome (MetS) that put us at risk for diseases such as type 2 diabetes, NAFLD, PCOS, cardiovascular disease, and metabolic-related cancers.

- Intermittent fasting treats the root cause of obesity, which is the high levels of insulin (hyperinsulinemia) that lead to insulin resistance. It helps our bodies to become insulin sensitive again.

How a Low-Carb, High-Fat Diet and Fasting Can Transform Your Health

. . . . .

"That temporary periods of undernutrition are helpful in the treatment of diabetes will probably be acknowledged by all after these two years of experience with fasting."
DR. ELLIOTT P. JOSLIN

W HEN I FIRST began to work with patients in the clinic, I would lead a six- to seven-hour training session to help them understand what intermittent fasting is and to get them into the right mindset to be receptive to this new approach. We talked a lot about food because what we eat is so important, and yet most people know very little about the effect on their body of the food they eat.

One question I always asked was "What five 'real' foods do you eliminate from your diet if you want to lose weight?" Take a moment to write down your answers now.

1 _____

2 _____

3 _____

4 _____

5 _____

My clients always mentioned the same foods: pasta, rice, bread, corn, and potatoes. *Every time.* Is that close to what you answered?

Did you know that *all* of those foods are low fat and low calorie?

Let's think about this a bit more. If current diets are right, then these are the foods you *should* be eating to lose weight. They're all low fat and low calorie, although most of us don't know that.

The obvious next question is "Why are you removing some of the lowest calorie and lowest fat foods from your diet?" My clients had no answer. Do you?

I loved this moment when patients started to put together how conventional advice was failing them. These conversations helped my clients see that it wasn't them who were failing; it was the diet industry. Two pervasive myths about food that impact those who are trying to lose weight and take a path to wellness are that dietary fat causes obesity and that eating small meals more often leads to weight loss. We looked at the second myth, *when to eat*, in the last chapter. Now I want to focus on *what to eat*.

We Are What We Eat

The old adage "We are what we eat" is true. Our bodies respond to the type of food that we consume by either increasing or lowering our insulin production. I want to take some time to look at each of the three basic building blocks of food, the macronutrients we call carbohydrates, protein, and fat. Each of these has a different function and causes a different hormonal response in the body. It's important that we understand how eating different foods impacts our insulin production.

Carbohydrates

Carbohydrates are foods like pasta, bread, potatoes, and grains. Whether they are whole grains like rice or refined ones like flour, carbohydrates often make up a large part of our diet. Some dairy products and fruit and vegetables also contain carbs, though in smaller amounts. The primary job in the body of carbohydrates is to provide food energy—think of carbohydrates as the body's main fuel source. Carbohydrates are split into two different types, which most of us have heard described at some point: simple and complex carbohydrates.

Simple carbs are made up of one or two sugar molecules, such as glucose and sucrose (combined these are table sugar). Common examples are candies, cookies, breads, pastas, and other foods made with lots of sugar or with refined grains (all flours and white rice, for example).

Complex carbs can be made up of hundreds or thousands of simple sugar molecules, and thus they are more complex in structure. Common examples are beans, quinoa, potatoes, sweet potatoes, and whole grains such as oatmeal and barley.

When we eat carbohydrates, the body breaks them down into their component sugars, primarily glucose, and signals the pancreas to release insulin. Remember, insulin is the key that opens the lock on cells so that glucose can get inside to provide energy. Insulin acts as the traffic controller directing the carbohydrates (sugars) to be energy for our cells. We need insulin to engage with an insulin receptor on the cell, which permits the glucose molecules entry inside. As we've already learned, insulin then directs any of this excess food fuel to be stored as glycogen reserves and then as fat to be used later.

Protein

Proteins are foods like meats, seafood, eggs, tofu, nuts, and seeds; made up of amino acids, proteins are a primary building block for growth and repair in the body. We only need so much protein for growth and repair, which comes as a shock to some of my clients because high protein is very trendy in the fitness and diet world right now. Despite what many commercials for protein powders or high-protein meal replacements would lead you to believe, eating a lot of protein doesn't make us or our muscles grow; it's *not* Miracle-Gro. Here's an analogy that will help you to understand why.

Imagine you're building a shed in your backyard. You only need so many bricks. If you order 10,000 bricks and only use 1,000 of them, then you have an excess 9,000 bricks you need to do something with. Consider bricks to be proteins, and this would be like a day you eat a lot of protein, as you've perhaps been told to do. That's a lot of extra bricks to have lying around. The body converts excess protein to glucose in the liver via a process called *gluconeogenesis*. This process causes our blood glucose levels to rise, which causes insulin to be secreted (but not a disease-causing amount) to get the glucose into cells. The body uses this glucose to fuel the body immediately or stores it to be used later when the body requires it. So, although protein can lead to the gluconeogenesis, protein itself is *not* really a fuel source. Your body only needs so much protein a day—you could eat 300 grams of protein, but your body maybe only needs 80 grams on that day for growth and repair. Your body will take the balance of protein (220 grams in this case) and convert it into glucose. If your body doesn't need that fuel immediately, then that glucose gets converted into body fat via insulin. That protein you're eating—those extra bricks—ends up on your body as fat.

Dietary fat

Dietary fat is found in foods like avocados, cheese and whole-fat dairy products, fatty fish, eggs, olives, and cold-pressed oils. This fat is made up of a glycerol backbone attached to fatty acids, and it's used to create new cells, healthy cholesterols, and many hormones and vitamins within the body. It can also be used to fuel the body. There are two main types of dietary fats: natural unprocessed fats and refined highly processed fats.

Natural unprocessed fats include omega-3s (fish), monounsaturated fats (olives, avocados, and their cold-pressed organic oils), and saturated fats (coconut fats such as coconut oil, butter, cream, and manna; full-fat milk; animal fats such as butter/ghee, leaf lard, bacon drippings, duck fat, and beef tallow). Often people label saturated fats as unhealthy and unnatural, but this isn't the case. Saturated fats are the basis of almost every cell in the body, and they are also a fuel source for the body. As saturated fat is a direct energy source, insulin secretion isn't triggered. Instead, fatty acids and ketone bodies are produced. Fatty acids fuel the body and ketone bodies fuel the brain.

• FATTY ACIDS AND KETONE BODIES •

When we need fuel while fasting, first we use our glycogen (stored glucose molecules). The body can store only so much glucose, so if you continue to fast after you've used your glycogen stores, your body needs to liberate fat from your fat stores to use as fuel. It does so via the process I mentioned earlier called de novo lipogenesis. Our body then produces free fatty acids and ketone bodies as fuel.

Free fatty acids provide most of the body's fuel when we fast. Ketone bodies are another source of fat fuels when you are in a fasted state. Fasting increases the number of ketone bodies we produce. When blood glucose or insulin levels are low, the body makes ketone bodies from fatty acids, which is a way for you to use up those stubborn fat stores and regain control of your body fat distribution. Unlike free fatty acids, ketone bodies can cross the blood-brain barrier to supply fuel for the brain.

There are three different types of ketone bodies: acetoacetate, acetone, and beta-hydroxybutyrate (BHB). BHB is the primary ketone body, and it's known to have anti-inflammatory properties. People with diseases of inflammation, such as rheumatoid arthritis, often follow a ketogenic diet high in dietary fat (and low in carbohydrates), so that they can produce ketone bodies to help reduce inflammation.

Refined highly processed fats include most seed and nut oils, such as vegetable oil, corn oil, canola oil, soybean oil, sunflower oil, and safflower oil. Have you ever squeezed the fat out of an olive? Easy to do. But what about a kernel of corn? Next to impossible. Extreme processing goes into extracting the fat from seeds and nuts, making these oils toxic for our body. Seed and nut oils create severe inflammation, which in turn triggers insulin secretion. (The only exception is macadamia nut oil, which is hard to find.)

We want to stick to naturally occurring fats as much as possible. Interestingly, if a naturally occurring food is *low* in fat, it will be *high* in carbohydrates, and vice versa.

- 1 gram of carbohydrate = 4 calories

- 1 gram of protein = 7 calories

- 1 gram of fat = 9 calories

All low-fat foods are naturally low calorie, but they break down into sugars, which trigger the release of the *most* fat-trapping hormone, insulin. What this means is that **we want to eat a diet higher in natural fats, moderate in proteins, and lower in carbohydrates**.

66

Eating for Optimal Health

Let me say it again. For optimal health, we want to eat a diet higher in natural fats, moderate in proteins, and lower in carbohydrates. I bet that surprises you, because it surprises my clients all the time. When I say they need to eat *more* natural fats, I can see their alarm. They think they are going to gain weight. My advice turns the food pyramid promoted by governments and many nutrition experts upside down, and that can be terrifying for people—especially women who've been bombarded with dieting advice since they were kids.

We now know that obesity is a disease of too much insulin (hyperinsulinemia), and we want to eat in a way that doesn't add more fuel to the fire. That means we don't want to add more insulin when we already have too much. Instead, we want to add healthy fats.

Not all calories are equal: The hormonal response

Conventional dietary advice assumes that all three macronutrients (carbs, proteins, and fats) evoke the same hormonal response in the body, but they don't. And we vilify dietary fat because 1 gram of fat has 9 calories. For reasons that don't make sense (which we looked at in Chapter 2), we believe that weight gain and loss is based on calories. But knowing that each macronutrient has a different function in the body, is it correct to assume they're all equal? The answer is no.

Dietary fat makes the body work harder to digest it, and therefore you spend more metabolic energy digesting fat than carbohydrates. Whether simple or complex, carbohydrates are very easy to digest and require extremely little metabolic energy to break down. Also, dietary fat doesn't require insulin to be produced in order to serve its various functions within the body. The free fatty acids that result when dietary fat breaks down can fuel most of our body and cross into cells without the assistance of insulin. Ketone bodies can cross the blood-brain barrier to provide most of the brain with fuel. Dietary fat does not trigger an insulin response because it doesn't need insulin to help get its food energy into cells.

In contrast, when we use glucose to fuel our cells, the body must produce insulin. Remember that insulin acts as a key that engages with the insulin receptor on a cell, allowing glucose to cross into it and provide energy. Protein provokes very little insulin response unless consumed in overly large quantities (at which point, as noted above, the excess protein is converted to glucose via gluconeogenesis in the liver).

If we consume more glucose than our cells need—whether from protein or from carbohydrates—our traffic controller, insulin, directs the excess glucose to be stored as glycogen (quick energy reserves in our liver and muscles). If those glycogen stores are filled up, insulin directs the excess glucose to be stored as fat (longer-term storage in our fat cells). This is where the misconception comes from that dietary fat and body fat are the same thing. That roll on your belly isn't a log of butter. It's excess glucose from too many potatoes, bread, or pasta dishes. While dietary fat and body fat are very different things, they share a name, and so dietary fat often gets blamed for the unwanted body fat you see reflected back to you in the mirror.

How would you answer now if I asked you, "Can we assume that 150 calories from a serving of almonds will have the same hormonal impact as 150 calories of soda?" The answer, of course, is no. These two foods may contain the same number of calories, but they have completely different roles in the body and entirely different hormonal responses. Let's explore this more.

Almonds are a combination of dietary fat, protein, and carbohydrates (mostly fiber). Dietary fat has many roles, and protein is primarily used for growth and repair. As the body breaks down almonds, very little insulin is produced, but quite a lot of metabolic energy is needed to digest them. In contrast, the soda is mostly water and all 150 calories are sugars. These sugars cause the body to secrete a significant amount of fat-trapping insulin very quickly after they're consumed, and the sugars can only be used for fuel.

Insulin resistance, SAD, and why fewer carbs and *more* fat are beneficial

When we follow the standard American diet (SAD), we're eating a diet that is low in natural fat and high in carbohydrates. We produce a lot of insulin in response to the high load of carbohydrates. Guidelines, especially for diabetics, ask us to eat three meals plus three snacks every day. If we do that, we're not only producing large quantities of insulin when we eat, we're also producing large quantities all the time! The result is toxic levels of insulin in the system (hyperinsulinemia). Over time, as we now know, hyperinsulinemia leads us to develop insulin resistance and the diseases associated with metabolic syndrome—such as obesity, high blood pressure (hypertension), high cholesterol, type 2 diabetes, and cardiovascular disease.

As we learned in Chapter 3, when we are insulin resistant, our insulin receptors no longer allow our own insulin to engage with them, and so glucose cannot enter our cells. This leaves an abundance of glucose circulating in the blood. The insulin converts what it can to glycogen but is forced to store the rest in fat cells, making them larger or even causing the body to produce extra fat cells for storage. The result is obesity and type 2 diabetes.

The reason many people lose weight and improve their blood sugar levels on a low carbohydrate, high healthy fat (LCHF) diet is that by eating fewer foods that break down into sugar, the body doesn't secrete as much insulin. In other words, the LCHF diet decreases the surges of insulin that overwhelm the body by decreasing the amount of carbohydrates, which break down into glucose, and by increasing the amount of natural fat, which crosses directly into the cells. Less insulin means less fat trapping. The

American Diabetes Association now recognizes the LCHF diet as a treatment protocol for type 2 diabetes. Following a LCHF diet helps us manage insulin secretion from *what we eat*. Intermittent fasting helps us manage insulin secretion based on *when we eat*. Together, they are a potent combination.

How Intermittent Fasting Is Different

Like me, I'm sure you've been inundated with advice on how to diet over the years. Perhaps you've tried shakes, meal substitutes, soup diets, point plans, or any number of other ways to try to lose weight. As we've explored, those diets all focus on Calories In versus Calories Out. But intermittent fasting is entirely different in six key ways. In the rest of this chapter, we'll explore each of these six ways so that you fully understand how intermittent fasting will be different from everything you've tried before.

1. Intermittent fasting treats the root cause of obesity by lowering insulin levels

Unlike other diets, intermittent fasting doesn't focus on Calories In versus Calories Out, or anything to do with calories. Instead, it treats the root cause of obesity, which is insulin resistance. The goal of intermittent fasting is to minimize the volume and frequency of insulin secretion in response to diet (what we eat). In addition to lowering insulin, intermittent fasting supports weight loss and optimal health in several important ways that calorie-restriction diets do not. This is because fasting triggers many hormonal adaptations that do not happen with simple caloric reduction. Three of these are very important to the health of your body:

1   Insulin drops precipitously, helping prevent insulin resistance.

2   Noradrenaline rises, keeping metabolism high.

3   Growth hormone rises, maintaining lean mass.

2. Intermittent fasting keeps resting metabolism high

Crucially, intermittent fasting prevents our resting metabolic rate (RMR) from falling. Several scientific studies prove this point. For example, over four days of continuous fasting, RMR did not drop in a study's participants.[1] It increased by 12 percent. Neither did exercise capacity decrease. Instead, it was maintained. Why does RMR remain stable or increase with fasting?

Imagine we are cavewomen. It's winter, and food is scarce. If our bodies go into "starvation mode," then we would have no energy to go out to find food. Each day the situation would worsen and eventually we'd die. The human species would have become extinct long ago if our bodies slowed down every time we didn't eat for a few hours. Instead, when we fast, the body opens up its ample supply of stored food—body fat! Resting metabolism stays high, and we change fuel sources from food to stored food (or body fat). We have enough energy to go out to hunt some woolly mammoth. Or in the case of a modern-day woman, perhaps we use that energy for work, family, or any of our other responsibilities.

During fasting, we first burn the glycogen stored in the liver. When that store is finished, we use body fat. Since there is plenty of fuel for most women in our body fat stores, there's no reason for our RMR to drop. We're not starving when we fast; we're fueling off our body fat. And that's the difference between long-term weight loss and a lifetime of frustrated dieting.

Fasting is effective where simple calorie reduction is not. What is the difference? *Obesity is a hormonal, not a caloric, imbalance.* Fasting provides beneficial hormonal changes. The hormonal changes that happen during fasting are entirely prevented when we eat constantly or go into starvation mode. So, it is the *intermittency* of the fasting that makes it so much more effective.

3. Intermittent fasting is consistent, not constant

Many calorie-reduction enthusiasts say that fasting works but only because it restricts calories. In essence, they are saying that only the average matters, not the frequency. Overall averages only tell us part of the story: for example, average national income doesn't highlight the income of a billionaire or of someone struggling to pay rent. Average days of sunshine won't let you know if today's going to be gray or cloudy. As soon as we start talking about calorie restriction, we assume that reducing 300 calories per day over one week will have the same effect as reducing 2,100 calories over a single day! The difference between the two is the knife edge between success and failure. Dr. Fung and I use the following analogy all the time. I share it with you here because it really helps clients visualize why we're advocating for an intermittent fasting protocol over calorie reduction as a primary strategy.

> Your eyes adjust whether you are in a dark room or bright sunlight. Your ears adjust if you are in a loud airport or a quiet house. The same applies to weight loss. Your body adapts to a constant diet by slowing its metabolism. Successful dieting requires an intermittent strategy, not a constant one. Restricting some foods all the time (portion control) differs from restricting all foods some of the time (intermittent fasting). This is the crucial difference between failure and success.
>
> **— DR. JASON FUNG**

4. Intermittent fasting breaks the cycle of persistent hyperinsulinemia

Conventional diet advice fails women because it doesn't look at our hormonal response to the food. The beneficial hormonal adaptations that occur during fasting are completely different from simple calorie restriction. And this is partly because intermittent fasting reduces insulin and insulin resistance. Insulin resistance depends not only on elevated levels of insulin in the body but also on those levels staying high. Intermittent fasting helps to prevent insulin resistance from developing because it keeps insulin levels low for extended periods of time.

Studies have directly compared daily caloric restriction with intermittent fasting, and kept the number of calories eaten during the week similar. A 30 percent fat Mediterranean-style diet with constant daily caloric restriction was compared to the same diet with severe restriction of calories on two days of the week.[2] Over six months, weight and body fat loss did not differ. But there were important hormonal differences between the two strategies. On the calorie-restricted diet, insulin levels, the key driver of insulin resistance and obesity in the longer term, fell initially but soon plateaued. However, on the intermittent fasting protocol, insulin levels continued to drop significantly. Insulin sensitivity improved with fasting only, despite the fact that both groups were eating a similar total number of calories. Since type 2 diabetes is a disease of hyperinsulinemia and insulin resistance, the intermittent fasting strategy succeeds where caloric restriction will not.

A second trial directly compared two weight-loss diets in obese adults.[3] The calorie-reduction model subtracted 400 calories per day from the estimated energy requirements of each participant in one group. The other group ate normally on eating days but ate zero calories every other day. In other words, they did an alternate-day fast (ADF). The study lasted twenty-four weeks.

The most important conclusion was that alternate-day fasting was a safe and effective therapy that anybody could reasonably follow. Both groups lost weight, and the fasting group did marginally better. This is consistent with most studies, where in the short term any decent diet results in weight loss. However, the devil is in the details. The fasting group lost almost twice as much fat around their trunk, which is the more dangerous fat around the organs. In fat mass percentage, the fasting group lost almost six times the amount of fat compared with the group following the calorie-reduced plan.

What happened to the participants' resting metabolism? This question is important because this is what determines long-term success. If you look at the change in resting metabolic rate between the two study groups, you can see the difference. Using the calorie-reduced diet, resting metabolism dropped by 76 calories per day. Using fasting, it only dropped 29 calories per day (which is not statistically significant compared to baseline). What this means is that during the study, daily caloric reduction caused almost 2.5 times as much metabolic slowdown as fasting. Although many women believe that fasting will put them into starvation mode, this study shows that intermittent fasting does the opposite.

5. Intermittent fasting does not increase hunger

If you've ever followed a calorie-restricted diet, you know that dieting makes you hungrier. The reason you find it hard to stop eating when you restrict calories is that ghrelin increases. Your body is telling you that it wants more food fuel to restore its energy balance. What's fascinating is that this hunger hormone goes up during calorie restriction but *not* during fasting. How hungry you are is not a matter of willpower; it's a hormonal fact of life—ghrelin goes up and you are hungrier. However, fasting does not increase hunger because it doesn't increase your ghrelin levels, and that makes it easier to keep weight off! You're less hungry, so you seek to eat less.

6. Intermittent fasting prevents weight regain

Fasting has a long history as a very effective way to control obesity. By contrast, the more recent daily calorie-restriction diets have been a stunning failure. The problem for most women who follow calorie-restriction diets is weight *regain*, not initial weight loss. A study comparing weight regain in one group following a calorie-restricted diet and a second group fasting found quite a difference.[4]

The fasting group tended to regain lean mass and continue to lose fat, whereas the calorie-restriction group regained both fat and lean mass. One interesting finding was that the fasting group reported they often continued to fast even after the study was done. They found intermittent fasting easier than they'd expected, and it produced better, longer-lasting results.

Compared with calorie-restricted diets, **intermittent fasting leads to more weight loss, more lean mass gain, more visceral fat loss, less hunger, lower insulin, and less insulin resistance**. Almost every medical society, doctor, dietician, and mainstream media outlet will advise you to follow a calorie-restricted diet. I prefer to tell people to fast intermittently.

Throughout these last four chapters, we've looked at the evidence that supports intermittent fasting and shared client stories to inspire you and get you excited about your own fasting journey.

Jana's Story

When I first met Jana, she was fifty-seven years old, stood 5 foot 2 inches, and weighed 177 pounds. Jana's doctor had diagnosed her with prediabetes, and her optometrist had noted that she was starting to show signs of eye damage related to diabetes. Jana was terrified of losing her vision.

Having heard from friends that a very low carbohydrate (ketogenic) diet might help her to lose weight and reduce her blood sugar levels, Jana had restricted her carbs to 25 grams per day. On her ketogenic diet, she had lost 60 pounds and improved her hemoglobin A1C reading, a measure of blood sugar levels, to 5.8 percent. But she had hit a plateau.

No matter how diligently Jana followed her ketogenic diet, she couldn't reduce her hemoglobin A1C results enough to be considered out of the prediabetic range and she wasn't able to lose any more weight. She became frustrated and came to see me to learn about fasting.

When we reviewed Jana's diet, it was evident she had made some wonderful changes. She had increased the amount of healthy fats she was eating and simultaneously reduced carbs. The problem was that Jana was grazing and snacking all day long, which was constantly stimulating her body to produce insulin. It wasn't about eating less, just less often, I told her.

To get a handle on her snacking, I suggested Jana save the almonds she usually ate as a snack at 9 a.m. and add them to her lunch around noon, and to save the cheese she often ate at 4 p.m. for her dinner later on. After she'd stopped snacking all the time, Jana began to eat two meals a day (TMAD). Her weight began to come down, and she was encouraged enough to eliminate all snacking and try fasting for 24 hours three times a week.

Within six months, Jana reached her goal weight of 130 pounds and stopped her prediabetes in its tracks. She continues to eat TMAD with the occasional 24-hour fast when it fits into her schedule. She feels great.

Now that you've heard Jana's story, you may be encouraged to begin your own fasting journey. While I understand that you want to fast right away to see how it works for you, it's important to understand how hormones other than insulin change our ability to succeed with our health goals. In the next part of the book, I focus on how those hormones impact our bodies.

We'll begin with a look at the impacts of stress and sleep on our bodies, learning how too much stress and too little sleep deeply affect your diet and your insulin and cortisol levels. After that, we'll spend time getting to know the hormones that are more specific to women, discovering how many of these interplay with female disorders.

My advice is that you take time with the next part of the book, much as you might want to leap into fasting right away. The more you understand the way your body works and how your hormones impact your entire system, the better able you will be to successfully meet your health goals.

Chapter 4 Takeaways

- The old adage "We are what we eat" is true. Our bodies respond to the type of food we consume by either increasing or lowering our insulin production. For example, 150 calories of soda provoke a very different hormonal response from 150 calories of nutritious food—one leads to obesity and disease, and the other doesn't.

- For optimal health, we need to eat a diet higher in natural fats, moderate in proteins, and lower in carbohydrates.

- Intermittent fasting is completely different from any other diet you've tried in the past because it is designed to lower insulin, not calories. There are six crucial differences between intermittent fasting and other diets.

- The goal of fasting is to minimize how much and how often the body secretes insulin in response to what we eat.

PART TWO

When Hormones Wreak Havoc:

How Intermittent Fasting Can Help Regulate Female Hormones

5

Cortisol
How Chronic Stress and Lack of Sleep Can Derail Weight and Fat Loss

. . . . .

*"When you have any ordinary ailment,
particularly of a feverish sort, eat nothing
at all during twenty-four hours. That will cure it.
It will cure the stubbornest cold in the head too.
No cold in the head can survive twenty-four
hours' unmodified starvation."*

MARK TWAIN

SOCIETY PLACES A lot of expectations on women. For many of us, juggling home care, childcare, and work responsibilities is extremely stressful. Short bursts of stress, what we call a rapid stress response, help us act quickly in times of emergency or reach a new goal. But chronic stress—stress that is constant and ongoing—wreaks havoc on our hormones and our bodies. And many of the medications used to treat conditions associated with stress, like anxiety and depression, contribute to obesity and metabolic syndrome. But, as we'll see in the following pages, until we can manage stress effectively, it's very difficult to experience the full benefits of intermittent fasting.

In this chapter, we'll look at cortisol, the hormone that's activated when we're stressed and when we don't get enough sleep. Many of us believe that we can skimp on sleep to fit everything else in, but we have to prioritize sleep in order to manage our hormones and our weight. We'll delve into the science of stress and its impacts, and then I'll offer some practical advice on how you can reduce stress in your life, using techniques such as meditation, exercise, and better sleep hygiene. The goal is to manage your cortisol levels so that you can set yourself up for intermittent fasting success.

What Is Cortisol?

Cortisol is a hormone we produce in response to stress. In Paleolithic times, this hormonal response was often to a physical stress, such as being chased by a predator. Cortisol prepared our bodies for action: to fight or flee. Today, there may be no mountain lions in the vicinity, but a stressful call with an employee; drama on the home front; caring for children, older relatives, pets, or friends; and perhaps volunteer obligations—often piling up at once—can all cause the same hormonal stress response. Whatever is stressing you, it raises your cortisol levels. Cortisol increases alertness and decreases the need for sleep. You know that feeling when your mind is spinning at the end of a long day? That's a sign of elevated cortisol levels.

As cortisol rises, glucose availability is substantially enhanced. The body draws on its emergency glycogen stores and breaks down proteins to convert them to glucose through gluconeogenesis. This glucose provides energy for muscles that are needed, say to avoid being eaten by that mountain lion chasing you down. At the same time, the body temporarily curtails its nonessential metabolic activities, such as digesting food and repairing damaged cells, to make all its energy available to survive the current and coming stressful period.

In our ancestors' times, soon after our cortisol levels rose, we would use up our newly available stores of glucose while fighting or fleeing the threat. Following this vigorous physical exertion, we were either dead, or the danger had passed. Our cortisol dropped back to a low level. Our bodies are well adapted to short-term increases in cortisol and glucose. But they are poorly adapted to chronic long-term stress. And many women now regularly experience chronic stress. For some, their cortisol levels remain elevated for months and years due to relentless stress and lack of sleep.

Cortisol raises insulin levels

At first glance, cortisol and insulin appear to have opposite effects. On the one hand, insulin, as we know, is a storage hormone. Under high insulin levels, the body stores energy as glycogen and fat. Cortisol, on the other hand, prepares the body for action. Our fight-or-flight response moves energy out of storage and into readily available forms such as glucose. That these hormones would have similar weight-gain effects seems unlikely. And indeed, with *short-term physical stress*, insulin and cortisol play opposite roles. But this situation is quite different for *long-term psychological stress*.

In modern times, chronic nonphysical stressors increase cortisol. For example, marital issues, problems at work, arguments with children, constant streams of text messages and emails, and sleep deprivation are all serious long-term stressors. Glucose flows into the body to prepare for a fight, but we don't vigorously exert ourselves physically afterward to lower blood glucose. Under conditions of chronic stress, glucose levels remain high. There is no vigorous physical exertion to burn off the glucose, and there is no resolution to the stressor, and so blood glucose can remain elevated for months. Chronic high levels of glucose triggers the release of insulin. And chronically elevated cortisol levels lead to increased insulin too. As you know from Chapter 3, hyperinsulinemia causes you to gain weight.

The Relationship Between Cortisol, Insulin, and Obesity

In the next two sections, we'll take a quick tour through the scientific evidence showing how cortisol and insulin interplay in the body and how impactful they are. What is important to understand is how cortisol levels (stress levels) affect your weight and how vital it is for stress reduction to be part of your overall wellness journey. So, let's begin.

As cortisol rises or falls, insulin follows

Using synthetic cortisol (prednisone), we can increase insulin experimentally. Healthy volunteers were given 50 milligrams of cortisol four times daily over five days. Insulin levels rose 36 percent from baseline.[1] Another study showed that the use of prednisone increases glucose levels by 6.5 percent and insulin levels by 20 percent.[2] Over time, insulin resistance also develops.[3] There is a direct dose-response relationship between cortisol and insulin. For every unit of free cortisol produced, the pancreas will produce ten times as much insulin.[4] In other words, long-term use of prednisone (synthetic cortisol) may lead to insulin resistance or full-blown type 2 diabetes.[5] Multiple studies confirm that increasing cortisol leads to insulin resistance.[6]

If cortisol raises insulin, then reducing cortisol should reduce insulin. And it does. In a study of transplant patients who were maintained on synthetic cortisol for years or decades as part of their antirejection medications, when they were weaned off the prednisone, their insulin levels dropped by 25 percent. This resulted in a 6.0 percent weight loss and a 7.7 percent decrease in waist girth.[7]

As you can see, the increased insulin caused by raised cortisol was harmful to health, in the same way that decreased cortisol and insulin helped reduced weight and girth.

Cortisol raises blood sugar where insulin lowers it. In a way, we should expect insulin resistance with cortisol because of this raised blood sugar causing insulin surges and therefore insulin resistance over time. And we know that insulin resistance leads directly to increased insulin levels (prediabetes) and obesity.

Cortisol causes weight gain and abdominal obesity

Does excess cortisol from long-term psychological stress lead to weight gain? Certainly anecdotal evidence seems to suggest that stress leads to obesity. But what does the scientific evidence say?

Studying patients with Cushing syndrome, a disease characterized by excessive cortisol production, helps demonstrate the impacts of cortisol on obesity. In 1912, brain surgeon Harvey Cushing originally described a twenty-three-year-old woman who suffered from weight gain, excessive hair growth, and loss of menstruation, giving a name to this disease. Since then, research has shown that up to a third of people with Cushing have high blood sugar levels and overt diabetes.[8] And patients who take prednisone or other similar corticoid medications for long periods often develop a particular redistribution of the fat from the limbs to the trunk and face called truncal obesity that is characteristic of people with Cushing.[9] The term *moon face* refers to a buildup of extra fat on the sides of the face. And a *buffalo hump* describes the fat deposited around the base of the neck between the shoulders. But the hallmark of this disease is weight gain.

Both cortisol and prednisone cause weight gain even in people without Cushing syndrome. Many patients complain that they gain weight no matter how little they eat and no matter how much they exercise. The ultimate test is this: Will somebody gain fat by taking prednisone? If the answer is yes, this proves a causal relationship rather than a mere association. Does prednisone cause obesity?

Absolutely! Weight gain is one of the most common and well-known side effects of the medication. High doses of prednisone causes weight gain. We raise cortisol; people gain weight. What all of this means is that **cortisol causes weight gain**.

Any disease that results in excess cortisol secretion results in weight gain. In a random sample of the general public from North Glasgow, Scotland, cortisol excretion rates were strongly correlated to body mass index (BMI) and waist measurements.[10] Heavier people had higher cortisol levels. Cortisol-related weight gain particularly deposits fat in the abdomen, which results in an increased waist-hip ratio (WHR). This weight distribution of fat in the abdomen is more dangerous to health than generalized fat because it surrounds our internal organs.

Cortisol may act through high insulin levels and insulin resistance, but so far this correlation is unclear from the research. There may be other pathways of obesity yet to be discovered. However, the fact that excess cortisol causes weight gain is undeniable. By extension, chronic stress causes weight gain. Many people have intuitively understood this connection despite the lack of rigorous evidence. It certainly makes sense. Much more sense than calories causing weight gain.

And what this means for you is that **reducing stress is vital in your weight-loss journey**.

Understanding Stress

Stress comes in two forms: emotional or physical. Most people associate emotional stress with negative emotions, such a death in the family or work pressure. But emotional stress can be negative or positive. Positive emotions, such as those associated with getting married or having a new baby, can cause stress responses in our body. I planned my own wedding, taking place in a different country than I was living in, and although the outcome was wonderful, the process was stressful. Moving into your dream home, getting a new pet, renovating your kitchen—all of these are stressful, even while joyful!

We might experience negative emotional stress if we're struggling with bad personal news, things feeling out of control, a divorce, a death, or negative global events such as a pandemic or war. Interestingly, the body responds the same way hormonally whether the emotional stress is positive or negative.

When we're in pain, we may have negative emotional stress, but we're also experiencing physical stress. Infections cause a stress response in the body, as does the flu, a broken bone, or a twisted ankle. And poor sleep causes an immense amount of stress in our bodies. We glorify busyness, but downtime is crucial for our bodies. We tell our friends that we're only getting five hours of sleep as if it's a good thing, but chronic poor sleep leads to chronic physical stress.

The difference between a rapid stress response and chronic stress is duration. What I see in a lot of my clients is a continuous stress response, one that never or rarely turns off. Their bodies have elevated cortisol, which makes managing hormones and weight extremely challenging. Reducing stress is difficult but crucial.

Contrary to popular practice, sitting in front of the television or computer is a poor way to relieve stress. Stress relief is an active process. Getting enough rest is one of the most important first steps.

The Connection Between Sleep Deprivation, Stress, and Obesity

One of the major causes of chronic stress today is sleep deprivation and disturbance. In 1910, people slept nine hours per day on average. By 1960, Americans were averaging 8.0 to 8.9 hours of sleep per night, and by 1995 that number had fallen further to seven hours. More than 30 percent of adults aged thirty to sixty-four report getting less than six hours of sleep.[11] Shift workers are especially prone to sleep deprivation and often report less than five hours of sleep. Many of my clients, especially women, take pride in how little they sleep. Sleep deprivation is not something to brag about. Even a single day of sleep deprivation can increase cortisol levels by over 100 percent.[12]

Lack of sleep leads to weight gain

Studies have consistently shown a relationship between short sleep duration, generally less than seven hours, and excess weight.[13] Cross-sectional studies from Spain, Japan, and the United States as well as longitudinal studies, such as the National Health and Nutrition Examination Survey (NHANES I) and the Women's Health Initiative, confirm this association.[14] The Quebec Family Study suggested a 27 percent increase in the risk of weight gain with shorter sleep duration.[15] A thirteen-year prospective study even suggested that every extra hour of sleep was associated with a 50 percent reduction in the risk of obesity.[16] A one-year prospective study showed that sleeping less than five hours per night was associated with a 91 percent increase in the risk of obesity. Sleeping five to six hours was associated with a 50 percent increased risk.[17] A meta-analysis of 696 studies published in 2008 showed that short sleep duration increased the risk of obesity by 55 percent in adults and 89 percent in children. For every hour of sleep deprivation, BMI rose by 0.35 kg/m².[18]

From a caloric expenditure perspective, this finding does not necessarily make sense. Sleeping less should increase energy expenditure since any waking activity uses more calories than sleep. Calorie theory would suggest that sleep deprivation leads to moving more and a lower likelihood of obesity. However, the opposite is true. Interestingly, sleeping more than eight hours per night may also increase the risk of obesity. The Western New York Health Study found that sleeping six to eight hours per night was associated with the lowest risk of obesity.[19] That study concluded that "excessive" sleeping—over eight hours—increased the risk of obesity by 60 percent, but too little sleep—fewer than six hours—*tripled* the risk.

Sleep deprivation raises blood glucose and insulin levels

Sleep deprivation is a potent psychological stressor. It stimulates cortisol, resulting in raised blood sugar; activates the sympathetic nervous system (our fight-or-flight response); and leads to both high insulin levels and insulin resistance. In one study, sleep deprivation resulted in 37 to 45 percent higher cortisol levels by the next evening.[20]

Researchers can measure the brain's glucose use through a type of imaging called positron emission tomography (PET). Glucose use by the brain decreases during sleep deprivation and likely contributes to the mental fogginess that we all experience when we're overtired. One study found that healthy glucose tolerance in volunteers who were restricted to four hours of sleep dropped by 40 percent. Their glucose response to breakfast was high enough to classify these previously normal individuals as having prediabetes! And their cortisol levels increased to close to 20 percent.[21]

Other studies have confirmed that it is possible to induce insulin resistance in healthy volunteers simply by restricting sleep to four hours per night, even for just one night.[22] After six days of sleep restriction, volunteers were 50 percent less insulin sensitive. In a Japanese study done with men, but still relevant to women in my clinical experience, shortened sleep duration increased the risk of type 2 diabetes.[23]

Lack of sleep leads to increased appetite

Both leptin and ghrelin, key hormones in the control of body fatness and appetite, are affected by sleep. Leptin increases steadily with more sleep. Higher leptin levels regulate body fat downward, making us thinner. Conversely, ghrelin, the hunger hormone, steadily falls with more sleep. Lower ghrelin means less hunger. The Quebec Family Study found that short sleep duration was associated with higher body weight, decreased leptin, and increased ghrelin.[24] Sleep deprivation of only four hours for two nights increased ghrelin by 28 percent and reduced leptin by 18 percent with accompanying increased hunger and appetite. Who can deny the late-night munchies? Many fast-food restaurants now cater to this phenomenon with twenty-four-hour service.

Interestingly, sleep deprivation under low-stress conditions does not decrease leptin or increase hunger.[25] This suggests that it is not the sleep loss that is harmful, but the fact that the disruption activates the stress hormones and hunger mechanisms.

What all this means concretely for you is that sleep deprivation will undermine any weight-loss efforts. Adequate sleep is not only essential to restore brain function but also to prevent the metabolic consequences of high cortisol and insulin resistance.

Stress and sleep deprivation form a vicious cycle

Sleep deprivation causes stress. But stress may also cause sleep deprivation. Increased cortisol or prednisone therapy, for instance, often causes insomnia because it activates the body's sympathetic nervous system, or fight-or-flight system. Patients often describe the sensation of having "too much energy." This is a classic vicious cycle. We see this cycle at work with obesity as well. Obesity can cause the problem of obstructive sleep apnea, where patients momentarily stop breathing during sleep. Repeated episodes of sleep apnea cause tremendous disruptions to normal sleep. This sleep deprivation then increases stress, which leads to more obesity.

An interesting natural experiment on sleep deprivation occurred in South Korea.[26] A 10 p.m. curfew was enforced on late-night tutoring schools. Follow-up surveys found that each one hour increase in sleep duration led to a 0.56 kg/m² reduction in BMI and a 4.3 percent reduction in obesity in the affected adolescents. In my clinical experience, the results apply to adult women too. When my clients incorporate sleep into their schedules and reduce stress, they see far better results in their bodies with their fasting plans.

Tips for Beating Stress and Getting More Sleep

You may already have your favorite way to manage stress. Maybe it's mindfulness meditation, yoga, massage therapy, or exercise. All of these are great, time-tested methods. Studies on mindfulness interventions used yoga, guided meditations, and group discussion to successfully reduce cortisol and abdominal fat.[27] But no matter which method you choose, I recommend that when you commence your fasting journey, you pick one and incorporate it. Don't make reducing stress a stressful activity! Pick one method for stress relief at a time. The one I like my clients to focus on first is increasing how much sleep they get: this lowers chronic stress and aids recovery.

· SIMPLE BUT EFFECTIVE WAYS TO IMPROVE SLEEP ·

- Sleep in complete darkness.

- Sleep in loose-fitting clothing.

- Keep your bedroom slightly cool.

- Keep all screens—TVs, laptops, phones—out of your bedroom. (This one can be hard, but clients who do follow it find themselves on a much more successful path to wellness.)

- Keep regular sleeping hours.

- Aim for seven to nine hours of sleep a night.

- See the light first thing in the morning—perhaps drink your coffee outside.

Lisa's Story

Lisa was struggling to lose weight and manage type 2 diabetes. When I first met her, she had recently lost her husband, was dealing with family issues, and was working as a cardiac nurse in an intensive care unit. When she started trying to fast, she realized that food was her best friend. She hung out with food when she was bored. She consoled herself with food as she grieved her husband. During stressful days at work, with hospital politics and dying patients, her only salve was food. This relationship with food made it difficult for her to fast and lose weight. She began to try out many different ways to reduce stress and incorporated meditation as her primary method.

Once she found the best way for her to reduce stress and increase sleep, her fasting became much more effective. So effective that she went from being a client to being a coach! She's lost 150 pounds and reversed her type 2 diabetes.

My wonderful colleague Lisa Chance has allowed me to share with you her list of thirty-nine ways to reduce stress and lower cortisol.

Thirty-Nine Ways to Lower Your Cortisol

1   Meditate.

2   Do yoga.

3   Stretch.

4   Practice tai chi.

5   Take a Pilates class.

6   Go for a labyrinth walk.

7   Get a massage.

8   Garden (lightly).

9   Dance to soothing, positive music.

10   Take up a hobby that is quiet and rewarding.

11   Color for pleasure.

12   Spend five minutes focusing on your breathing.

13   Follow a consistent sleep schedule.

14   Listen to relaxing music.

15   Spend time laughing and having fun with someone. (No food or drink involved.)

16   Interact with a pet. (It also lowers their cortisol level.)

17   Learn to recognize stressful thinking and begin to:

   • Train yourself to be aware of your thoughts, breathing, heart rate, and other signs of tension to recognize stress when it begins.

   • Focus on being aware of your mental and physical states, so that you can become an objective observer of your stressful thoughts instead of a victim of them.

   • Recognize stressful thoughts so that you can formulate a conscious and deliberate reaction to them. A study of forty-three women in a mindfulness-based program showed that the ability to describe and articulate stress was linked to a lower cortisol response.[28]

18   Develop faith and participate in prayer.

19 Perform acts of kindness.

20 Forgive someone. Even (or especially?) yourself.

21 Practice mindfulness, especially when you eat.

22 Drink black and green tea.

23 Eat probiotic and prebiotic foods. Probiotics are friendly, symbiotic bacteria in foods such as yogurt, sauerkraut, and kimchi. Prebiotics, such as soluble fiber, provide food for these bacteria. (Be sure they are sugar-free!)

24 Take fish or krill oil.

25 Make a gratitude list.

26 Take magnesium.

27 Try ashwagandha, an Asian herbal supplement used in traditional medicine to treat anxiety and help people adapt to stress.

28 Get bright sunlight or exposure to a lightbox within an hour of waking up (great for fighting seasonal affective disorder as well).

29 Avoid blue light at night by wearing orange or amber glasses if using electronics after dark. (Some sunglasses work.) Use lamps with orange bulbs (such as salt lamps) in each room, instead of turning on bright overhead lights, after dark.

30 Maintain healthy relationships.

31 Let go of guilt.

32 Drink water! Stay hydrated! Dehydration increases cortisol.

33 Try emotional freedom technique, a tapping strategy meant to reduce stress and activate the parasympathetic nervous system (our rest-and-digest system).

34 Have an acupuncture treatment.

35 Go forest bathing (shinrin-yoku): visit a forest and breathe its air.

36 Listen to binaural beats.

37 Use a grounding mat, or go out into the garden barefoot.

38 Sit in a rocking chair; the soothing motion is similar to the movement in utero.

39 To make your cortisol fluctuate (which is what you want it to do), end your shower or bath with a minute (or three) under cold water.

— LISA CHANCE

Women especially tend to juggle many roles in their lives, and I find that many of my clients are stressed and fatigued. Understanding how difficult it is to lose weight when cortisol is elevated is helpful to many of my clients, and I hope that you are able to reduce your own cortisol levels as you move forward with the book.

Cortisol is not the only hormone that can wreak havoc in the body. Next, we'll look at estrogen, a hormone that causes problems for many women when it becomes dominant.

Chapter 5 Takeaways

- Stress takes both physical and emotional forms, and whether it's positive or negative, it raises cortisol levels.

- Higher cortisol levels are associated with high insulin levels and fat gain.

- Lack of sleep raises cortisol levels hugely.

- Reducing stress and increasing sleep are two ways you can improve your chance of success with intermittent fasting.

- There are many ways to lower cortisol, and I recommend everyone try different methods, one at a time, until they find what works for them.

Female Sex Hormones, Part 1
How Estrogen Dominance Disrupts Menstruation and Metabolism

· · · · ·

"She who eats until she is sick must fast until she is well."
ENGLISH PROVERB

FEMALE HORMONES IMPACT all of our bodily systems, and it's important to understand how. This chapter covers a little bit more about what hormones are and how the key female hormones act in your body, before we focus on estrogen. It's crucial to think about this hormone specifically because so many women struggle with symptoms of estrogen dominance. If you recognize yourself in this chapter, this information will help as you progress through your fasting journey, strengthening your mindset and guiding you as you set healing goals.

Let's start with the absolute basics. I want to share with you everything I know, and everything I've learned clinically and personally so that you have the most up-to-date and helpful information.

Female Hormones 101

Hormones, such as cortisol and insulin, are chemicals that work as messengers in the body. Think of your hormones as car drivers. They carry messages around the body in the most efficient way, following the most efficient route—just like an Uber driver does!

Our endocrine glands, which are all over our body, secrete these chemicals so that hormonal messages can be sent throughout the body to control our physical and emotional selves. Here are some examples of how hormones regulate our bodies:

- Height is tightly regulated by human growth hormone.

- Bone turnover is tightly regulated by parathyroid hormone.

- Blood sugars are tightly regulated by insulin and glucagon, among others.

- Reproductive systems are tightly regulated by testosterone and estrogen.

The list goes on and on. Any bodily function you can imagine is under some regulatory system—and that is usually hormonal (endocrine, paracrine, autocrine, and so on).

Our hormones need to be in the right balance for our bodies to work optimally. All hormones get metabolized in our liver, meaning they get broken down into their inactive and active parts. Sometimes those inactive parts can be toxic for the body. The liver's job is to try to neutralize the toxic substances produced during this metabolism. Some genetic factors and nutrient deficiencies make it hard for the liver to do its job, and the toxic substance stays in the body. This metabolism is therefore critical to good health, and when it isn't working well, it leads to hormonal imbalances.

When our hormones are in balance, we don't think about them because our body works efficiently, and we feel great. When our hormones fall out of balance, however, we feel sluggish; we can't conceive; and we exacerbate existing health conditions or develop new ones. Our imbalanced hormones force us to pay attention to our body. Many of the health issues we deal with as cisgender women are due to hormonal imbalances, particularly imbalances that affect our sex hormones. Most women experience symptoms of hormonal imbalance at some point. Some of these symptoms, such as headaches, acne, or brain fog, are relatively common. Here's a partial list of other common issues related to an imbalance of female sex hormones, many of which you may recognize:

- weight fluctuation

- gastrointestinal issues, such as abdominal pain, diarrhea, vomiting, and constipation

- infertility

- irregular periods

- low sex drive

- mental health issues

- mood swings

- poor sleep quality

- unstable blood sugar

- vaginal dryness

- breast cancer

Managing weight through intermittent fasting is a key part of balancing our hormones to improve and prevent many conditions, including the two most common: estrogen dominance and polycystic ovary syndrome.

Before we look at what happens when our hormones are out of balance, it's useful to know a little bit about each of the female sex hormones: what they do, and how they impact the body. We'll start with estrogen and progesterone, the two hormones women are often most familiar with, then we'll quickly travel through the four other (less recognized) female sex hormones.

Estrogen: Estradiol, estriol, and estrone

Estrogen is one of the two hormones that women associate with their menstrual cycle. There are actually three types of estrogen in the body, and the main one is estradiol. In the first part of the menstrual cycle, estradiol levels rise, causing an egg to mature and be released and thickening the uterus's lining, ready for that egg to implant.

Estradiol is the most important of the three forms of estrogen women produce. It is mainly produced by our ovaries, and when in balance, estradiol makes us feel great. (When it is out of balance, it can cause a lot of problems.) It prevents us from developing insulin resistance and gaining weight, and it's protective against cardiovascular disease. It can alleviate symptoms of anxiety and depression. During the first two weeks of our menstrual cycle when estradiol is high, we feel invincible and like a sexy superstar. As with all hormones, too much can be problematic, and too little makes us feel down and insecure. Mood swings, for example, are often the result of a fluctuation of this hormone, along with high progesterone. As we enter menopause, our bodies don't produce as much estradiol. Our adrenal glands, the tiny glands above our kidneys that make cortisol and produce our sex hormones, help to offset the decline by producing another form of estrogen called estrone (which we'll look at in a moment).

Estriol is the second of the three forms of estrogen that women naturally produce. Normally the body makes it only in very small amounts, but starting about the eighth week of pregnancy, the placenta makes estriol in larger amounts and keeps producing it until the baby is born. Otherwise, it's fairly insignificant in terms of its role.

Estrone, the third of the three forms of estrogen that women produce, is made by our fat cells and adrenal glands. As we enter menopause and our body produces less estradiol, estrone becomes the predominant form of estrogen in the body. Obese women tend to produce more estrone from their fat tissues, and too much estrone can contribute to growths (fibroids) and cancer (endometrial cancer). It can also cause significant problems when it is being metabolized in the liver.

Estrogen metabolism is critical and can be a significant predictor for how we age. We'll look at the various pathways to metabolize estrogen later in this chapter.

Progesterone

Progesterone is made predominantly in the ovary during the second half of the menstrual cycle. When an egg is released from the ovary at ovulation, what's left of the follicle that enclosed the egg becomes the corpus luteum and it releases progesterone. To prepare the body for pregnancy if the egg is fertilized, progesterone levels rise. Progesterone trims the endometrial lining that was thickened thanks to estrogen's influence. These two hormones work in a balancing partnership to stop the lining of the uterus from becoming too thick, which can lead to cancer. As we age, however, progesterone production goes down, and we lose this balance.

If the egg isn't fertilized, the corpus luteum breaks down, progesterone levels fall, and a new menstrual cycle begins. Progesterone helps to regulate ovulation and has an impact on mood. It's known as the fun, sleepy hormone or sometimes as the pregnancy

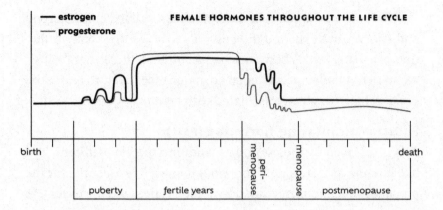

hormone because it helps create ideal conditions for the fetus to grow. Progesterone is key to hormone replacement therapy, which has been a controversial therapeutic path.[1]

Low progesterone is associated with menstrual irregularity, appetite changes, low libido, hot flashes, migraines, depression, anxiety, and other mood fluctuations. Many women have trouble falling asleep as they age because they don't produce enough progesterone. My mother-in-law, for example, struggled to sleep more than three hours a night. Six months ago, she started to take bioidentical progesterone supplements (which is not the same as hormone replacement therapy), and now she's sleeping full nights, has lost weight, and has her hormones in balance.

Dehydroepiandrosterone (DHEA)

DHEA is made almost exclusively by the adrenal gland (although a smaller amount is made in the ovaries). DHEA is a precursor hormone and weak androgen, which means that it has little effect on its own but becomes powerful when converted to other hormones, such as testosterone or estrogen. It mostly converts to androstenedione, which then converts to testosterone or estrogen. DHEA peaks in our twenties and thirties, with a slow decline expected with age. This hormone produces about 75 percent of estrogens before menopause and 100 percent after.

This hormone appears in urine as DHEA sulfate, androsterone, and etiocholanolone, and the best way to assess the total production of DHEA in the body is to add up these three metabolites. When DHEA is elevated, women are much more likely to have acne or facial hair, which are associated with PCOS.

Follicle-stimulating hormone (FSH)

FSH is released by the pituitary gland into the bloodstream, and like luteinizing hormone (more on it below), it is essential for the proper development and function of the ovaries (and the testes). In the first part of the menstrual cycle, FSH stimulates the follicles in the ovary to grow. Similar to the partnership between estradiol and progesterone, the balance between LH and FSH is key. Around day eighteen of the menstrual cycle, if LH is too much higher than FSH, then the body will not release an egg. Women with PCOS have this hormonal imbalance, which prevents them from releasing an egg at the right time.

Luteinizing hormone (LH)

This hormone is released by the pituitary gland, and it is important for regulating how the ovaries (and the testes) work. In the first part of the menstrual cycle, LH stimulates the follicles in the ovary to produce estradiol. It then triggers the release of an egg from the ovary (ovulation). After ovulation, LH stimulates the corpus luteum to release progesterone to support pregnancy. Luteinizing hormone plays a critical role in maintaining fertility, and so this hormone is key for people with PCOS. LH works in synergy with follicle-stimulating hormone (FSH) to stimulate follicular growth and ovulation.

Testosterone

We think about testosterone as a male hormone, yet it is produced in both the ovaries and the adrenal gland. Testosterone is a precursor to estradiol, and it regulates the secretion of LH and FSH. Testosterone levels normally decline with age. Perimenopausal testosterone levels can increase before declining again. If women have low free testosterone, they can't build muscle—which increases the risk of age-related health issues since we lose the ability to produce it as we get older. Too much testosterone in women can lead to acne and hirsutism and is associated with PCOS.

Estrogen Dominance

Estrogen plays an important role for women, and not just for our reproductive systems. Estrogen contributes to bone health, protects our cardiovascular system, and influences our mood and behavior. Too much estrogen can lead to several forms of cancer, as well as PCOS, premenstrual syndrome, and endometriosis. Although our genetics play a part in how our body produces and metabolizes estrogen, our lifestyle has an effect too. And how estrogen is metabolized is more important than most of us realize. At some point in her life, virtually every woman in North America suffers from estrogen dominance.

High body fat and high stress both contribute to elevated estrogen levels, as can taking some medications such as birth control pills, drinking too much alcohol, or doing anything that compromises proper liver function. Let's take a look at the two main reasons estrogen levels can be high: your body is producing too much estrogen (or not enough progesterone to keep it in balance), or your body is not breaking down estrogen and removing it.

Estrogen dominance and the menstrual cycle

The first half of the menstrual cycle is known as the follicular phase. In the ovaries, small sacs of fluid known as follicles begin to grow because estrogen levels are starting to rise. Each of these follicles has the potential to release an egg. Just before ovulation, estrogen spikes, causing luteinizing hormone (LH) to release from the pituitary gland and stimulating the primary follicle to release the

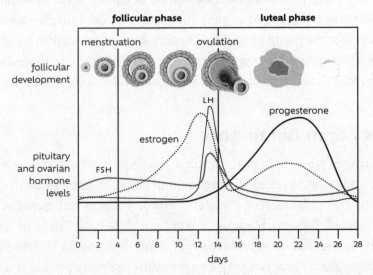

THE MENSTRUAL CYCLE

egg. This release is known as ovulation and typically occurs midway through the cycle. The second half of the cycle is known as the luteal phase. After the egg is released, the leftover follicle closes, becomes known as the corpus luteum, and starts to produce progesterone. If an egg is not fertilized and an embryo implanted in the uterus, the hormones fall, and the body sheds the uterine lining in the menstrual period.

If you do not ovulate or do not ovulate very well, your progesterone levels are not healthy, which reduces your chances of implantation and increases the risk for miscarriage. If your estrogen is not healthy, you may not stimulate the LH surge needed to prompt ovulation, which means you're then not releasing an egg.

Common estrogen dominant symptoms associated with the menstrual cycle include breast tenderness, mood swings, and heavy bleeding. If you do not metabolize estrogen properly, it may indicate a bigger issue with folate, which is critical to fetal development. A test that reveals your hormone pattern throughout the month may show abnormal rises, falls, or flatline levels.

Jasmyn's Story

Jasmyn was twenty-one years old and had not menstruated in three years when she showed up to her consultation with her mother. While Jasmyn wasn't sure if she wanted to be a mom one day, her own mother wanted to make sure Jasmyn had that choice. Jasmyn wasn't concerned about her health, but her mother was so frustrated and upset about Jasmyn's lack of menstruation that it had led to constant fights. I suspected that estrogen dominance might be the reason that Jasmyn wasn't menstruating.

When her mom left us alone to chat, Jasmyn and I talked about her lifestyle and what she might change. She was not willing to adjust her diet. She worked at a fast-food restaurant and enjoyed eating out with friends. She struggled to buy higher quality food due to high tuition fees and cost of living. We agreed that she would commit to fasting three times a week for 42 hours each time. On the other two days, she would eat twice and cut out all snacking between those two meals.

Three months later, Jasmyn had her period. In the following months, she continued to menstruate about every twenty-eight days. Even so, Jasmyn continued her 42-hour fasts three times a week for eighteen months before moving to a two meal a day (TMAD) protocol.

Several years later, Jasmyn came to see me again because she had started to gain weight. She still had a normal period, but she couldn't lose the extra weight easily. She began the longer fasts again, using the same protocol as before, but this time she also ate a moderate low-carb diet (50 to 100 grams of carbohydrates each day). Within a year, she was back to a healthy weight, and her migraines, which are a common symptom of estrogen dominance, had subsided.

Today, Jasmyn continues to eat two low carbohydrate, high healthy fat meals a day to manage her weight and her menstruation.

Estrogen dominance and metabolism

We metabolize estrogen in the liver, using a two-phase process to detoxify and excrete it. Phase one is called *hydroxylation*. When estrogen breaks down, it's toxic. Adding a single oxygen and a single hydrogen molecule to the estrogen—hydroxylation—makes it non-toxic. During this stage, enzymes break down estrogen using one of three different pathways. Each pathway describes the placement of the oxygen and hydrogen molecules on the estrogen, which you can think of as parking spots. The first pathway is the 2-OH (2-hydroxy) pathway. If the oxygen and hydrogen are parked in the 2-OH spot, it's the right parking spot: the pathway to paradise. Everything that follows this path can be properly metabolized—meaning that all of the toxic properties can be neutralized and the resulting metabolites are estrogenically inactive. We want all three estrogens to go through *this* pathway, and when they do, we feel great.

But there are two other pathways where things start to go wrong. Not such good parking spots! The 4-OH (4-hydroxy) pathway is bad news. Estrogen that uses this pathway does not completely break down. The resulting estrogen metabolites are still partly active and can damage your DNA, leading to certain types of tissue growth and cancers. The 16α-OH (16α-hydroxy) pathway is worse news; like the 4-OH pathway, estrogen that uses this pathway does not break down completely and can lead to growths like fibroids, growths, polyps, and cancers.

Phase two of estrogen metabolism involves two parts. The first part is called *methylation*. Both the 2-OH and 4-OH involve this step, which further detoxifies (or in the case of the 2-OH pathway creates beneficial) estrogen metabolites. Metabolites from the 16α-OH do not undergo methylation and therefore remain more active. The second part of phase two is called *glucuronidation*, and in this stage metabolites from all three pathways are mixed with glucuronic acid and excreted from the body.

The bottom line is that if estrogen isn't leaving the body through the 2-OH pathway, then the remaining toxins lead to estrogen dominance. Weight gain, high cortisol due to stress, and alcohol all lead to increasing estrogen. So, too, does age. As our menstrual cycle ceases and our body naturally stops producing progesterone, our estrogen levels can get too high. And in addition to the growths and cancers noted above, estrogen dominance can also result in insulin resistance.

How we metabolize estrogen is largely genetically determined. Unfortunately, we can't control whether our body breaks down estrogen through the 2-OH, 4-OH, or 16α-OH pathway. Which is all the more reason to eat a low carb, high healthy fat diet and fast intermittently. When we use these tools to keep our weight in check and our insulin low, we limit the growth environment for the cancers, fibroids, and polyps that the toxins in our estrogen metabolites can breed.

How to Determine and Rebalance Your Estrogen Levels and Metabolites

Estrogen metabolites can't be measured in a regular blood test, although you can check your levels of estradiol, estriol, and estrone that way. To test how your body is metabolizing estrogen, you need to take a Dried Urine Test for Comprehensive Hormones (DUTCH analysis) by Precision Analytical, or a SpectraCell test. Be reassured that many women have this problem of poor methylation, and it is a very important factor in predicting our longevity. Nutrient deficiencies are also a result of poor methylation. People who are poor or so-so methylators, and even those who are good methylators but growing older, are at risk of early death and disease.

If you discover that your body is metabolizing estrogen along a poor pathway, there are supplements to push estrogen down the 2-OH pathway: glutathione and n-acetyl cysteine (NAC). Both are amino acids that act as antioxidants to help to prevent and repair cell damage. Vitamins B_{12} and B_6 as well as choline (which you find in eggs or organ meats like beef liver) are also extremely important nutrients to support estrogen metabolism.

Losing weight, reducing stress, and reducing alcohol consumption are all key to managing estrogen dominance. And fasting is an effective way to help you lose weight and also reduce your insulin secretion, which helps you manage your estrogen dominance. But even if you manage your weight, meditate three times a day, and don't drink a lot, aging puts this hormonal balance at risk.

Once you reach menopause, taking bioidentical progesterone supplements to keep your body and progesterone and estrogen in balance is my advice. *Bioidentical* means that the hormones are derived from plant or animal sources and are chemically identical to the ones your body produces. They are different from the synthetic hormones used in traditional hormone replacement therapy, which our bodies failed to recognize. Remember the Women's Health Initiative study we looked at earlier? Women in this study who took synthetic hormones had all sorts of disease risk increase, especially breast and ovarian cancers. Bioidentical hormones do not carry this risk. I have taken bioidentical progesterone myself and highly recommend it.

In this chapter, we've taken time to get to know our female sex hormones and we've looked in more detail at what happens when estrogen becomes dominant. Next, I want us to look at PCOS, a disease that many women struggle with and that merits special attention because it's so common. Understanding its root causes and symptoms has helped many of my clients succeed on their fasting journey.

Chapter 6 Takeaways

- Our hormones carry messages throughout our body, and they need to work in balance for our body to perform optimally.

- We have several female sex hormones, which carry messages to begin and regulate our menstrual cycle. The levels of our female sex hormones change throughout our menstrual cycle and throughout our lives.

- When our hormones are not in balance, we suffer from many symptoms. Learning these symptoms is the first step in managing our health.

- Estrogen plays an important role for women, and not just for our reproductive systems. Many women are estrogen dominant, and intermittent fasting can help manage excess weight and insulin secretion, which contribute to hormonal imbalances. Using bioidentical supplements can also help.

7

Female Sex Hormones, Part 2

How Too Much Insulin Can Lead to Elevated Testosterone and Polycystic Ovary Syndrome

• • • • •

"To lengthen thy life, lessen thy meals."
BENJAMIN FRANKLIN

POLYCYSTIC OVARY SYNDROME (PCOS) has only been considered a disease in the last century, but it is actually an ancient disorder. Originally described as a gynecological curiosity, PCOS is now the most common endocrine disorder in young women, and it is known to involve multiple organ systems. In this chapter, we'll look at how our understanding of PCOS has evolved, how it is diagnosed, and how and why a low carbohydrate, high healthy fat diet and intermittent fasting can help reverse both the symptoms and the disease.

Understanding PCOS

Hippocrates (460–377 BCE), the father of modern medicine, first described "women whose menstruation is less than three days or is meagre, are robust, with a healthy complexion and a masculine appearance; yet they are not concerned about bearing children nor do they become pregnant." This early description of PCOS existed not only in ancient Greece, but in ancient medical texts around the world. Scientists throughout history continued to note women with similar "mannish" attributes, and the eighteenth-century Italian scientist Antonio Vallisneri connected these masculinizing features with the abnormal shape of the ovaries into a single disease. He described several young infertile peasant women whose ovaries were shiny with a white surface and were the size of pigeon eggs.[1] By the 1920s, scientists had started to call these symptoms a syndrome, named Achard-Thiers.

The modern era of PCOS began in 1935 when Drs. Irving Stein and Michael Leventhal made the connection between the lack of menstruation and the presence of enlarged ovaries. They coined the name *polycystic ovary syndrome* to describe a lack of menstruation, enlarged ovaries, and masculine features. This disease was originally thought to have been caused by female fetuses having too much exposure to androgens, but this hypothesis was ultimately refuted in the 1980s. Instead, studies have increasingly linked PCOS with insulin resistance and hyperinsulinemia.[2] The prefix *hyper-* means *too much*, and the suffix *-emia* means *in the blood*, so the word *hyperinsulinemia* literally means "too much insulin in the blood." I like to think of PCOS as the type 2 diabetes of the ovaries. Research linking PCOS to insulin resistance has paved the way for us to regain control of our bodies by lowering our insulin levels through intermittent fasting.

How to Diagnose PCOS

At the second international conference on PCOS held in Rotterdam, the Netherlands, in 2003, PCOS was recognized to represent a *spectrum* of disease. In other words, not all symptoms appear in all patients. It was decided that at least two of the following symptoms needed to be confirmed for PCOS to be diagnosed.

1 **Hyperandrogenism:** Male sex hormones, called androgens, are usually present in both males and females. The best-known androgen is testosterone. Many women with PCOS have elevated androgen levels, with associated symptoms such as increased body and facial hair growth (hirsutism), male-pattern baldness, acne, low voice, and menstrual irregularities.

2 **Anovulation or oligo-ovulation:** Many women with PCOS have rare or irregular menstrual periods or none at all. These menstrual irregularities are caused by the failure to ovulate. *Anovulation* means that no egg is released from the ovary. *Oligo-ovulation* means that few eggs are released. This difficulty ovulating results in difficulty conceiving and infertility.

3 **Polycystic ovaries:** The Rotterdam criteria defined polycystic ovaries as the presence of twelve or more follicles measuring 2 to 9 millimeters in diameter in each ovary. More recently, that number has been revised to twenty or more.[3] During normal menstruation, many follicles begin to develop with one eventually becoming the egg that is released into the uterus at the time of ovulation; the other follicles shrivel up and are reabsorbed into the body. When these follicles fail to shrivel up, they become cystic—full of liquid—and are visible on an ultrasound as ovarian cysts.

These three criteria are now used to diagnose PCOS. It is important to note that although obesity, insulin resistance, and type 2 diabetes are often associated with PCOS, they are not diagnostic criteria. PCOS should not be considered lightly, however. It is associated with a number of reproductive and metabolic diseases, including the top two causes of death in America: cardiovascular disease and cancer.

· WHEN WHAT LOOKS LIKE PCOS IS NOT... ·

Hyperandrogenism and polycystic ovaries are not exclusive to PCOS, so other diseases that resemble PCOS must be ruled out. While these conditions are rare, they can be serious and require entirely different treatments, so making the distinction is important. The list of similar conditions includes:

- pregnancy

- prolactin excess

- thyroid disease

- adrenal hyperplasia

- Cushing syndrome

- androgen-producing tumors

- drug-induced androgen excess

PCOS can only be diagnosed when these other problems have been excluded by history or a physical or laboratory examination.

The Connection Between PCOS and Reproductive and Metabolic Disorders

PCOS is not merely a nuisance: it is an important warning. The overall economic burden of PCOS in the United States is shocking: the cost of diagnosing and treating PCOS in women aged between fourteen and forty-four years has been estimated at $4.37 billion annually.[4] This amount is three times the cost of treating hepatitis C. A full 40.5 percent of that cost comes from treating the related condition of type 2 diabetes. Even more sobering, this number is likely a severe underestimate of the true costs, since it only takes into account the reproductive years and not postmenopausal problems. Complications arising from type 2 diabetes, heart attacks, strokes, and cancer—all higher risks for women with PCOS—typically happen in the postmenopausal years and are much more expensive to treat.

PCOS and reproductive concerns

Dr. John Nestler, chair of the Department of Internal Medicine at Virginia Commonwealth University, estimates that "if a woman has fewer than eight menstrual periods a year on a chronic basis, she probably has a 50 to 80 percent chance of having polycystic ovary syndrome based on that single observation."[5] An estimated 85 percent of women with PCOS suffer from menstrual irregularities.[6] The lack of ovulation makes it difficult to conceive, and PCOS is the most common cause of infertility in industrialized nations. The disease is also associated with recurrent miscarriages, fetal concerns, and gestational diabetes.[7]

INFERTILITY

If you don't ovulate, you can't conceive. Although women with PCOS usually have difficulty conceiving, rather than are infertile, the possibility of infertility can cause severe anxiety. Anovulatory cycles, most due to PCOS, account for approximately 30 percent of visits to an infertility clinic. The Australian Longitudinal Study on Women's Health, a community-based survey of young women, found that a heartbreaking 72 percent of women with PCOS considered themselves infertile, compared to only 16 percent of women without PCOS. The use of fertility hormones in the PCOS group was almost double that of the non-PCOS group. The 5.8 percent of women identified as having PCOS made up a whopping 40 percent of those seeking fertility treatments.[8]

Medications such as clomiphene have been relatively successful at inducing ovulation and helping women get pregnant. However, these treatments often have serious side effects—physical, psychological, and financial.

MISCARRIAGES AND OTHER PREGNANCY-RELATED COMPLICATIONS

Losing a pregnancy can be absolutely devastating, especially if it was difficult to conceive in the first place. Miscarriage, also known as spontaneous abortion, occurs in an estimated one-third of women with PCOS.[9] The root cause of PCOS is hyperinsulinemia, and elevated levels of insulin can cause higher levels of luteinizing hormone (LH). Excess LH generates more androgens. And this hyperandrogenic environment in the ovary often leads to miscarriage.

Rates of all pregnancy-related complications are increased in women with PCOS.[10] Gestational diabetes, pregnancy-induced hypertension, and pre-eclampsia risks are approximately tripled. Risk of preterm birth is increased by an estimated 75 percent when compared to women without PCOS or those who have overcome PCOS. Women with PCOS are also more likely to deliver by cesarean section, which itself comes with complications. Many of these complications are due to high insulin levels and obesity.

Many women with PCOS undergo fertility treatment to help with conception. These fertility treatments may double the risk of multiple pregnancies and the complications that come with them.

FETAL CONCERNS

Mothers with PCOS have a higher risk of small-for-gestational-age babies as well as babies that are large for their gestational age. Twin births, for example, have up to ten times the risk of being small-for-gestational age and a sixfold risk of premature delivery. Mothers with diabetes commonly have larger babies, whether they suffer from PCOS or not, likely because hyperinsulinemia increases the amount of nutrients available to the fetus. Both small and large sizes are associated with metabolic complications later in life (type 2 diabetes, obesity, and hypertension),[11] admissions to the neonatal intensive care unit, stillbirths, and perinatal mortality.[12] Hyperinsulinemia in utero may possibly affect the child's intellectual and psychomotor development as well.

GESTATIONAL DIABETES

Women with PCOS, particularly if they are obese, have about twice the incidence of gestational diabetes (GD) of women without PCOS. Higher insulin resistance is associated with gestational diabetes, which increases the future risk of type 2 diabetes, cardiovascular disease, and metabolic syndrome. Gestational diabetes also increases the risk of miscarriage, delivery by cesarean section, or induced birth due to the larger fetus. Maternal obesity increases the risk of childhood obesity and PCOS.

PCOS AND ASSOCIATED HEALTH CONDITIONS

PCOS significantly increases the risk of developing metabolic syndrome and other serious diseases related to hyperinsulinemia and insulin resistance. Aside from type 2 diabetes, among the most common associated health conditions are endometrial and ovarian cancers, cardiovascular disease, and nonalcoholic fatty liver disease.

CANCER

Women with PCOS are three times more likely to develop endometrial cancer when compared to the general population.[13] Ovarian cancer is also increased two- to threefold. Since there is a significant overlap between hyperinsulinemia, obesity, and PCOS, it is no surprise that women with PCOS are also at higher risk of the cancers associated with overweight and obesity, which make up 40 percent of all cancers diagnosed in the United States.[14]

CARDIOVASCULAR DISEASE

PCOS's overlap with metabolic syndrome means that women with PCOS may be at risk of cardiovascular disease. Some studies estimate a sevenfold increase in risk over women without PCOS.[15] Since cardiovascular disease is already the leading cause of death in older women, this finding is especially concerning.

DEPRESSION AND ANXIETY

Depression and anxiety are associated with PCOS but not necessarily caused by it. In my clinical experience, a lot of women are upset about the symptoms they experience, which lowers their self-esteem. Male-pattern and excessive hair growth, acne, obesity, and menstrual irregularities can destroy self-esteem, especially during adolescence, which may be one of the reasons that depression, anxiety, and other psychological problems are increasing among younger women with PCOS.[16] Infertility may also provoke feelings of inadequacy that lead to depression. Chronic illnesses associated with PCOS—such as type 2 diabetes, cardiovascular disease, and cancer—may cause depression too.

DIABETES/METABOLIC SYNDROME

The disease most closely associated with PCOS is type 2 diabetes, which is part of the metabolic syndrome along with obesity. Approximately 82 percent of women with type 2 diabetes have multiple cysts on their ovaries, and 26.7 percent fulfill the criteria for PCOS.[17]

Women with PCOS have three times the risk of developing type 2 diabetes by menopause when compared to the rest of the population. By age forty, up to 40 percent of women with PCOS will have already developed type 2 diabetes. In a group of women with PCOS, 23 to 35 percent will have prediabetes and 4 to 10 percent will have frank type 2 diabetes.[18] This rate of prediabetes is three times higher, and the rate of undiagnosed type 2 diabetes is 7.5- to 10-fold higher than women without PCOS. PCOS is recognized by the American Diabetes Association as a risk factor for diabetes.

People being treated for type 1 diabetes are also at risk of PCOS. An estimated 18.8 to 40.5 percent are affected, compared to only 2.6 percent in the control group.[19]

NONALCOHOLIC FATTY LIVER (NAFLD)

This disease of fat accumulation in the liver of a patient who consumes little alcohol is the most common form of liver disease in the Western world. NAFLD affects an estimated 20 percent of the general population worldwide, but about 75 percent of those with type 2 diabetes.[20] The connection between NAFLD and PCOS has only emerged since 2005. Since then, many studies have confirmed the tight correlation between the two diseases. Women with PCOS are 2.5 times more likely to develop NAFLD when compared to women without PCOS.[21] NAFLD is often underdiagnosed because the disease has practically no symptoms and is really only discovered through blood tests. Approximately 30 percent of women with PCOS have evidence of liver damage show up their blood tests. Fifty to 80 percent of women of reproductive age investigated for NAFLD also had PCOS.[22] In my clinical experience, it's important to screen for this condition. The good news is that fasting is very effective at reversing NAFLD. I've transformed my own NAFLD through intermittent fasting protocols.

SLEEP APNEA

Obstructive sleep apnea (OSA) is a condition where the upper airway collapses during sleep. People with sleep apnea cannot breathe for an instant, which leads them to briefly wake up, though they usually don't remember it the next day. When this happens throughout the night, their regular sleep patterns are disrupted. The main symptoms of this disease include snoring and excessive daytime sleepiness. Like NAFLD, OSA is highly linked to metabolic syndrome and obesity. The rate of OSA in women with PCOS is an astounding five to thirty times higher than women without PCOS.[23]

How Hyperinsulinemia and Insulin Resistance Lead to PCOS

Although obesity, insulin resistance, and type 2 diabetes are commonly found along with PCOS, they are *not* part of the diagnostic criteria. In my clinical experience and in the research literature, though, evidence does point to obesity or insulin resistance as the root cause. Take the following case report as an example.[24] A twenty-four-year-old woman was admitted to the hospital with unusual symptoms. During exercise, she had experienced a grand mal seizure, without any previous history of epilepsy. In the prior six months, she had become very tired and noted episodes of trembling, blurred vision, and confusion. She could control these symptoms by eating something.

Upon investigation, she was found to suffer from a rare insulin-secreting tumor of the pancreas known as an insulinoma. This tumor was massively overproducing insulin, causing her blood sugar to fall very low—as low as 1.6 mmol/L after an overnight fast. She had way too much insulin in her body. She also noted that she had acne and hirsutism and that her periods had become very irregular, from forty- to forty-four-day cycles over the previous year. An ultrasound revealed polycystic ovaries, and bloodwork revealed high testosterone levels, which gave her a diagnosis of PCOS. She had a normal body mass index and was not overweight.

After surgery to remove the two-centimeter tumor in her pancreas, her symptoms resolved. Four months after her successful operation, her menstrual cycles regulated to twenty-eight days, she lost 4 kilograms (8.8 pounds), and her acne and hirsutism fully resolved. Bloodwork revealed that her insulin level had normalized and, along with it, her testosterone levels.

This story shows just how closely excessive insulin and PCOS as well as weight gain are connected, which is one of many reasons why I believe that PCOS must be considered more than just a disorder of excess facial hair, acne, and fertility issues. The close link to obesity and type 2 diabetes suggests that all three conditions have the same underlying root cause. All three are now considered metabolic diseases, which means that all three conditions have the same underlying problem. That problem is hyperinsulinemia.

High insulin impacts the ovaries

Studies have confirmed that high insulin increases androgen levels. Direct insulin infusion measurably increases the levels of androgens: what this means is that the more insulin you have, the higher the testosterone production in your ovaries.[25]

The ovary is particularly rich in insulin receptors, which may seem strange at first glance because insulin is a hormone most commonly associated with digestion, blood glucose, and body fat. Why would the ovaries carry insulin receptors? The answer is that both pregnancy and raising children require a lot of resources, including enough food for both the mother and the developing fetus. All mammals need to know that food is available before they commit to reproduction. When you eat food, insulin rises, which is a signal that energy resources are available. The ovary's insulin receptors pick up this fact and proceed to develop and release eggs normally.

We know that adults can survive on relatively low levels of food energy and nutrients. During World War II, for example, many people lived on what would now be considered woefully inadequate amounts of food. Because our adult bodies are no longer growing—our bones and internal organs remain the same size—we can maintain regular cell function by breaking down old worn-out cells to build new ones, a process known as autophagy. A fetus, however, needs enough nutrients to build and grow internal organs, muscles, proteins, fat cells, and so on. Although a person might weigh only 7 pounds at birth, they might eventually grow to 150 pounds or more—and that growth requires nutrients. The ovary must therefore have reliable information about how much food is available in the outside world so that it releases eggs only when it is abundant. The ovary relies on nutrient sensors to provide that information. And insulin is one of the ovary's nutrient sensors.

Remember how we looked at the impact of insulin resistance and the trigger of constant stimulation? It seems that this stimulation causes metabolic illness and also increases testosterone. Increased testosterone leads to the development of acne and hirsutism in PCOS.

High insulin arrests follicular development

As we saw in the last chapter, the ovaries contain a number of follicles that, under normal circumstances, grow and release an egg each month. High insulin levels disturb the delicate balance of follicle-stimulating hormone (FSH) to luteinizing hormone (LH) that triggers correct follicular development, which can lead to anovulation or oligo-ovulation, as well as polycystic ovaries.[26] During normal ovulation, a surge of LH selects one of these follicles—the primary follicle—to mature and release an egg. However, the high insulin levels associated with PCOS make all of the follicles too sensitive to LH. The small follicles stop growing, no single dominant follicle is selected, and no mature egg is released. Furthermore, the follicles do not receive the message to close up, shrink, and be reabsorbed by the body. This means that the many small follicles accumulate fluid and become cystic. These numerous small fluid-filled cysts are visible on ultrasound and clinch the diagnosis of PCOS. The reason for the development of polycystic ovaries is follicular arrest, which is ultimately caused by too much insulin.

With PCOS, the high levels of insulin send a "stop growing" message to the follicles too early. As a result, too many follicles do not mature to become eggs. These immature follicles cannot be expelled as eggs (and pushed out to the uterus for fertilization) and they never shrivel up either, and so there is a failure of ovulation. This failure of ovulation causes menstrual irregularities.

Too much insulin leads to both the cysts and the overabundance of testosterone that causes hyperandrogenism in PCOS.

How to Reduce Excessive Insulin and Testosterone and Reverse PCOS

We tend to believe that increased growth is always good, but in truth **growth in adults is almost always bad**—apart from pregnancy and breastfeeding. Excessive growth is the hallmark of cancer, for example. Excessive growth leads to more scarring and fibrosis. Excessive growth of cysts leads to polycystic kidney disease and polycystic ovary syndrome (PCOS). Excessive growth in adults tends to be horizontal, not vertical. In most cases of adult disease, we want less growth, not more. And one of the best ways to restrict uncontrolled growth is by managing our nutrient intake. When we lower our insulin levels and fast intermittently, we do just that.

We know that PCOS is a disease of excessive growth, and in women of reproductive age, the most rapidly growing cells are in the ovaries. In women of reproductive age with PCOS, high insulin levels in the body encourage excessive growth, particularly cysts in the ovaries. Strategies that reduce insulin, like fasting and eating a low carbohydrate, high healthy fat diet, lead to weight loss and also reverse PCOS in many cases. That's certainly what I've seen with my clients over and over.

Melissa's Story

Melissa had never had a regular period in her life. Since her first period when she was eighteen years old, she'd never had a period more than once a year. In addition to these menstrual irregularities, she had some acne and male-pattern hair growth. And she had always been overweight. Her oligo-ovulation and hyperandrogenism meant she met the diagnostic criteria for PCOS.

Melissa wanted to have children. But after three unsuccessful rounds of in vitro fertilization (IVF), she gave up on the idea of conceiving a child of her own. She and her husband adopted a child, Luka. Melissa's period still only came once a year, and she knew she was at increased risk of developing cancer and other complications associated with PCOS. Cancer ran in her family: both Melissa's dad and paternal aunt had had breast cancer, as well as both her grandmothers—and she worried about developing the disease in the future.

Melissa began to work with my Fasting Method colleague Nadia Pateguana to cut out all refined carbs and sugars from her diet and to incorporate intermittent fasting into her lifestyle. Melissa lost some weight, and her periods started to come every forty-five days. Her doctor did some follow-up tests. Knowing that Melissa and her husband wanted to have more children, the doctor encouraged them to do one more round of IVF. "You might just ovulate," the doctor said.

In 2009, Melissa got pregnant through IVF. Her pregnancy was very healthy, and she gave birth to Sam when Luka was 2.5 years old. She never had blood sugar or blood pressure concerns. She lost more weight after having Sam and breastfeeding him for two years. Afterward, her menstrual cycle started to come regularly every thirty-two days.

Melissa and her husband thought their family was complete. He booked a vasectomy. Just before the surgery, Melissa found out she was pregnant! She had another very healthy pregnancy, and Mikha was born in 2013. Melissa is now the mother of three, and she has managed to maintain her low-carb diet, adjusting as needed to keep her menstrual cycle regular and prevent the risks associated with PCOS.

As we've seen in these last three chapters, hormones play a powerful role in our bodies. When we understand this, we also better understand why lifestyle changes can make a difference physically and emotionally. The science we've covered in these last chapters will help you understand why a low carbohydrate, high healthy fat diet and intermittent fasting can help you lose weight, regulate your hormones, reverse many metabolic diseases, and improve your overall health both in the short and the long term.

Next, I want to share what I've learned—through my own experience and helping others—about how to introduce and maintain these lifestyle changes successfully. These are the practical tips, tricks, and tools to motivate you as you begin and to help you through the tough times. Let's get started!

Chapter 7 Takeaways

- Doctors have described the symptoms of PCOS since ancient times, but only in the modern era has it been described as a spectrum of disease.

- Many symptoms are associated with PCOS, but the three diagnostic criteria are hyperandrogenism, polycystic ovaries, and anovulation or oligo-ovulation.

- Scientific research shows a connection between elevated levels of insulin and testosterone and the symptoms of PCOS.

- PCOS is a disease of too much growth, as are other metabolic diseases. Adult women can manage this excessive growth through intermittent fasting.

PART THREE

Fasting for Optimal Health: How to, When to, and Tips for Troubleshooting

8

Prepare to Fast
Build a Healing Mindset and Cut Out Snacks

• • • • •

"The best of all medicines is resting and fasting."
BENJAMIN FRANKLIN

KNOWING WHY A low carbohydrate, high healthy fat (LCHF) diet and intermittent fasting can benefit your health is one thing. Knowing how to fast safely and effectively is another. Remember that when I first started fasting, I jumped in with both feet and ended up hungry and exhausted. So, whether you've read the previous chapters and are excited to move forward with your fasting intentions or have jumped straight to this section (I do recommend taking time with the earlier parts of the book), I want to guide you step by step through introducing intermittent fasting into your lifestyle, just as I do when working with a new client.

In this chapter, I'll help you prepare to fast and give you some tools to incorporate your new eating plan into your life, so your transition to fasting is as easy as possible.

Fasting has become very popular in the past ten years. You've probably seen the word *fasting* plastered across the cover of magazines, heard people talk about fasting, or followed a favorite celebrity on their fasting journey. If fasting had been as widespread when I began as it is now, I would have found all the information overwhelming. The focus of this chapter is to cut through that overwhelm to make fasting a reality for you. We'll go over what to consider before you start your first fast, some important rules for fasting, and strategies to keep you feeling well through your first fast.

Take a Step-by-Step Approach

Fasting is like a muscle that you need to train. If you begin strength training at the gym, you don't expect to start with the same program that a body builder would use. We have to start where we're at, and weightlifting is hard. So, the way that we get stronger is that we start with 10 pounds, then add 10 more pounds, until we feel more comfortable with what we're lifting. If you follow this step-by-step approach and work at it, perhaps you'll be able to squat your own body weight.

We understand this progression when it comes to going to the gym. The same progression is true with fasting. Each of us needs to start from a comfortable place and make adjustments. Just as physiological adaptations happen when we start weightlifting, when we fast for the first time, we learn to navigate a new normal—otherwise known as behavioral change—and manage hunger.

Changing behavior

Fasting is a change in behavior. Some clients come to me when they are eating eighteen times a day: from the moment they get up to the time they go to bed. A step-by-step approach to fasting allows you to change those eating behaviors gradually so that you aren't going from zero to a hundred overnight. For example, after your first few days of building your fasting muscle, a small behavioral change might be that you see donuts at work, but you don't reach for them. Learning how to fast, step by step, helps with the mental adjustment while simultaneously reducing our insulin secretion, which reduces our insulin resistance. Slow and steady is effective, and it's prevented so many of my clients from falling into a cycle of deprivation and reward. I'd love for you to try this approach with me.

Managing hunger

The less often we eat, the less we want to eat because we are not constantly stimulating insulin. And when we stop secreting insulin constantly, we don't produce the hunger hormone, ghrelin, as frequently, which means we don't feel as hungry. This slow and steady approach to fasting has a gradual effect on our hunger hormones and satiation signaling.

Learning anything new takes time. In this and the next chapter, we're going to look at four steps—building a healing mindset, cutting out snacking, using fat fasting, and dropping one meal a day—that will help you transition from your current eating practice to a healthy and effective intermittent fasting practice. These steps could take you a few weeks to practice, or maybe longer. The process and the timeline are very individual, but I recommend you spend at least a day or two on the focused work of getting into the right mindset. Spend two weeks learning to cut out snacks, and then two more weeks on dropping one meal. Fat fasting is an option that some people use if they have trouble adjusting at any of the steps, and some people use fat fasting as a distinct step. Other people don't use it at all. As you move forward, please know that this journey is designed as a path for you to follow, and you're invited to go faster or slower depending on your body and on the advice of your doctor.

Usually when I work one on one with clients, we find the best timeline for their busy lives. I recommend that you think about your timeline too. Look at what's in your calendar—and avoid starting this journey when you have an upcoming vacation or very stressful period at work. Think about how long you will spend building your mindset and how long you might spend on steps two and three, before you contemplate the fasts explored in the next chapter.

Before you begin any of these steps, keep in mind these tried and tested rules for fasting.

· RULES OF FASTING ·

1   Do not fast if you are pregnant or breastfeeding.

Fasting is antigrowth, and pregnancy is a period of growth in the body. Fasting is *not* advised when you're pregnant because that growth is important for your body and the health of your child. Similarly, fasting is not advised when you're breastfeeding because it interferes with the quantity and quality of your breast milk.

2   Do not fast if you are malnourished.

Our bodies are made up of 10 to 13 percent essential fat, and the range for healthy body fat for an adult woman depends on age. Body composition is very important to people who live a fasting lifestyle, as we explore in the final chapters of this book. For the moment, it's important to know that a body with less than 18 percent body fat is considered malnourished, and fasting is not advised if your body fat level is this low. If you do not know your body fat level but suspect you are at the low end, you can find out your exact percentage by doing a body composition analysis, also known as a DEXA scan (see Chapter 13).

3   Check with your doctor before fasting.

Intermittent fasting is safe and effective when done properly. Before you make any nutritional change, check with your doctor and be sure to have them follow you on your fasting journey.

Fasting can lower your blood sugar levels and your blood pressure, which can be life-threatening in some situations. It's essential that a doctor monitor you if:

- You're on medication. You can't stop your medications all at once! A doctor may need to adjust dosages or the medications themselves, and they must monitor you until you reach a stage of wellness where you are able to contemplate ceasing medication.

- You have or are at risk of hypoglycemia (low blood glucose) or hypotension (low blood pressure). Both conditions can be life-threatening and your doctor needs to monitor both, as do you, while you fast.

Some doctors are unaware of the benefits of fasting and may be uncomfortable supporting you through fasting. It's extremely important that you find a medical ally on your journey. Resources such as LowCarbUSA.org and DietDoctor.com can help you find a supportive in-person doctor in the United States and other countries around the world.

4   If you have a history of disordered eating, seek clinical guidance before you fast.

A history of disordered eating doesn't prevent you from fasting, but you should check with your doctor first. If you have a history of anorexia, bulimia, or body dysmorphia, for example, it's essential that you work with a psychologist or a psychiatrist to see if fasting could ever be right for you. Key to our Fasting Method team is our behavioral psychologist, and she helps people manage their disordered eating, care for their emotional and psychological responses around eating, and learn how to have a strong and healthy relationship with food. For example, someone who binges on cookies will learn from our behavioral psychologist how to break that habit. Be sure that you work with a clinician *before* you begin any fast.

5 Stop your fast anytime you feel unwell or uncertain.
When you do anything for the first time, you may experience some discomfort, but you should not feel ill when you fast. Many people ask me how to recognize that line of feeling unwell, and I always answer that they need to stop fasting when they feel *uncertain*. Trust your instincts if you're feeling unsure, and check in with a clinician. You can always fast another day.

If your body sends you any of the following red flags when you're fasting, *stop your fast immediately* and check in with your doctor:

- nausea

- flu-like symptoms

- a drop in your (measured) blood glucose level that makes you feel uncertain

If you stop fasting—and while you wait to consult with a doctor—you can stick to time-restricted eating (page 154) and avoid unhealthy foods. This approach will keep you on a path to wellness until a doctor has reviewed your situation.

Now that you've reviewed the rules of fasting, it's time to work through the first step on your fasting journey: prepare for intermittent fasting through behavioral change. First, set your mindset, and then cut out snacking.

Learning to Fast, Step One: Build a Healing Mindset

Many people associate fasting with feelings of deprivation. They have thoughts like, *My family is having dinner, and I'm not joining them. He's having a cookie, and I'm not.* I recommend that you change how you look at a fasting day to help you get into the right state of mind.

Some yoga teachers start their classes by asking participants to set an intention, and that works for fasting as well. What is it you want to achieve with your fasting journey? In a moment, I'll ask you to list your goals. But first I have a crucial distinction for you: instead of *deprivation*, I want you to think about *healing*. When we teach ourselves from the outset that we're healing our bodies by fasting, it helps us shift our mindset. I think of fasting as my treatment, because it transformed my health.

Write a list of healing goals

With this idea in mind, take a moment now to help your mind reframe the work you're about to do for your body. Write a list of all the healing things you're hoping to achieve by fasting. For example,

- lower blood sugar levels

- improve thyroid function

- increase fertility

- _____

- _____

- _____

- _____

- _____

- _____

- _____

Look at the healing goals you want to achieve. Picture yourself attaining each of these goals. Are there others you'd like to add? When your list is complete, copy your list of healing goals and carry it around with you, or pin it to your bathroom mirror. Whenever you get caught up in feelings of deprivation, look at your list of healing goals and remind yourself that you're on a path to wellness.

Use wellness language

Our thoughts are the language of our mind. Over time, our recurring thoughts become beliefs and guide the way we see the world. Our feelings are the language of our body. To change how we feel, we have to change our thoughts and beliefs. The words we use are powerful tools of change. Just as I want you to focus on healing rather than deprivation, I want you to think about rebuilding rather than eating. So, our fasting days are *healing* days, and our eating days are *rebuilding* days.

To succeed at fasting, leave the language of *deprivation*, *reward*, and *indulgence* at the door. In our current lifestyle, food has become our best friend: we hang out with it, console ourselves with it. When we're fasting, we can't use the language of *indulge* or *reward* for eating days because it confuses our already complicated relationships with food. When we reframe what we choose to eat on our rebuilding days, we don't indulge with soda and cookies. We want to rebuild with natural fats and nutrients. Using the language of healing and rebuilding helps us to do that.

Learning to Fast, Step Two: Cut Out Snacking

Nowadays, we eat constantly. Our phones and TVs display a steady stream of ads for takeout foods and quick snacks, our nutritional guides often advise six small meals a day, and our workplaces build in coffee breaks every three to four hours. But it hasn't always been this way.

Cutting out snacking begins to extend our healing window, flex our fasting muscle, and demonstrate the potential health benefits of intermittent fasting.

No snacking is better for our physical health

On *Leave It to Beaver* (a popular 1950s and '60s TV sitcom), the youngest son, Beaver, always wants to eat. He wants a snack before dinner or more ice cream before bed. His mom, June Cleaver, says no every time. It's the one North American pop culture staple that discouraged snacking in favor of three meals a day—*and no more*.

When I first started fasting, my family found the idea challenging to understand, except for my grandmother. I remember her saying, "It wasn't until we started snacking that we gained weight. Nobody got sick until we started snacking. When your dad was growing up, we didn't have snack food. Your dad didn't go to school with snacks to consume all day long; it was just different in those days. We had three meals. That's it." She remembered a time before snacking became a part of our day-to-day existence. Just like June Cleaver, my grandmother believed in three meals a day—*and no more*. I mention this story because knowing that snacking isn't how people have always eaten helps us challenge the notion that it's "normal."

Cutting out snacks reduces our cognitive load

Even if you've always had snacks as part of your daily eating plan, consider that cutting out snacks reduces cognitive load. What does that mean? The more decisions we have to make, the more we increase our cognitive load—the mental strain we place on our brains to process and synthesize information. When we choose not to snack, we don't have to revisit that question several times a day when a snack is offered or available, and we don't have to decide what or when to eat between meals. Reducing cognitive load is healthy for everyone, but especially for anyone who is feeling overly busy or stressed.

Skipping snacks is a great stepping stone to time-restricted eating

As we change our behavior by cutting out snacks, we begin to see the possibilities for building more healing periods into our day. And we start to see the wellness benefits that result. Among my patients, I see a *lot* of disease prevention through this step. I see reductions in inflammation levels, insulin resistance, and conditions such as type 2 diabetes and PCOS that are caused by insulin resistance. Inspired to try this step yourself? Try cutting out snacks for one day. Then see if you can manage it for two days. Slowly build up more days in a row, like you would if you were lifting weights at the gym.

For some women, cutting out snacks is all they want to do. It's the perfect wellness path for the time of life they're in because it gives them control over their health choices, reduces inflammation, and prevents weight gain. And the magic of cutting out snacks is that, when you're ready, you can ease into a 14-hour fast without having to change very much in your life at all. If you eat breakfast at 8 a.m. and finish dinner at 6 p.m.—and you don't snack before or after those times (or preferably during that time window either)— you have 14 hours between the last meal of the day and the first one in the morning. You've moved yourself into a 14-hour fast without changing anything in your life other than refusing snacks.

If you're healthy and you want to maintain good health, a 14-hour daily fast (time-restricted eating) might be right for you. It can also be a great strategy once you've regained your health with one of the longer fasting protocols. A 14-hour-a-day fast won't cure disease, but it will get you one step closer to wellness.

Saying no to snacking trains us to deal with challenges

Many women, especially mothers, struggle to balance work, family, driving kids everywhere, attending evening meetings, and managing the household. And many women, mothers or not, struggle with fitting in a proper time window to eat. Grabbing a snack on the run often seems easier than cooking a meal—and it often seems preferable when the kids are picky eaters, everyone is eating at different times, you have back-to-back meetings, or you don't feel like cooking. But while those snacks seem like a quick solution to hunger, as we know they cause long-term health issues. If you can resist the urge to snack—or to replace meals with snacks—then you are training your body to adjust to the physiological progression of fasting.

As you begin to cut out snacking, you will encounter some challenges that test you mentally—and you will need to draw on your healing mindset to deal with them. Snacking cues are everywhere. When you pass cafés and fast-food restaurants and hear and see ads for food all day long, and yet you resist snacking, you train your mind and body to ignore conditioned responses to food. All of us have normalized snacking: we're habituated to snacks after school, during movies, while driving.

When your friends and family prompt you to eat with them or express surprise or concern when you no longer snack (or go ahead and munch *their* snacks), you'll learn to remind yourself how cutting out snacks is helping you meet your healing goals.

We are used to fueling before we feel hungry. When we're used to snacking, we can feel hungry when we don't actually need food. It's important to remember that hunger doesn't get worse and worse; instead, like a wave, it peaks and then passes. This knowledge is powerful because it helps you to have the patience you need to ride the wave.

Here are two other tips to help train you to ride the hunger wave. If you find it hard to avoid snacking when you're cued or habituated, change *where* you are. For example, if you're in the kitchen while others are snacking, could you leave the room or the house? Often hunger is exacerbated by thirst. If you're feeling hungry, try drinking green tea, water, or coffee to feel satiated.

Consistency Is Key

Remember that consistency is the foundation of successful intermittent fasting, and that is especially true for women. Weight loss is more complicated for women because we're much more hormonally complex than men. But that doesn't mean we can't get the same results. We *can* get the same results. We just follow a different pathway. Whereas men tend to lose a lot of weight when they begin to fast, that weight loss then slows down. For example, a man can lose 10 pounds during Week 1, but then only 1 or 2 pounds on Week 12—and some weeks he may not lose any weight at all as his body tries to dump the more stubborn fat.

What we see in women is the total opposite. Women are slow to start, with little or no weight loss some weeks. But with patience and consistency in their fasting protocols, their weight loss starts to pick up! A woman may not lose any weight on Week 1, but she may lose several pounds during Week 12.

I've seen many women throw in the towel after a few weeks because they think intermittent fasting is just another dietary fad that won't work for them. As a formerly obese woman who has tried almost every diet on the planet myself, I get it. But nothing worthwhile comes easily. Life is a nonstop roller coaster: one day everything is going well, and the next day your world comes crashing down. And what have we been taught to do when that happens? Comfort ourselves with food. If you're a woman looking to lose weight at pretty much any stage of life, you need to nip this reaction in the bud right now. We face bumps and hurdles almost every day. But if you stick to your fasting—unless you have a reason to stop following the rules of fasting—you will get results.

As you prepare for your first fast, build a strong healing mindset and use what you learn from cutting out snacks or trying a 14-hour fast to develop consistency and resilience. My whole life, I've watched patients and loved ones yo-yo between weight gain and weight loss, and I spent the first twenty-seven years of my life yo-yoing between a healthy lifestyle and falling off the wagon completely. And because of the type 2 diabetes, fatty liver, and PCOS that resulted, I had to be real with myself when I committed to fasting.

I had the option to try to hit my goals by ditching fasting when I was stressed out about work, angry at my husband, or sad that my grandmother died. And that option would have meant dealing with the damage type 2 diabetes was doing to my body. My second option was to fully commit to my fasting protocol 90 percent of the time for six months. Anything less would put me in the yo-yo category. Anything more wasn't human. I had to permit myself to slip up occasionally but not let one bad food choice turn into a day or week of bad choices. A firm commitment meant I could set a healing goal to kick my obesity, type 2 diabetes, PCOS, and fatty liver in six months and move on with my life. Reaching that goal was slow as hell to start, but nothing that truly works comes easily. Consistency was the key, and as you know, in six months I reached every part of my healing goal.

Halle's Story

Halle was in her late fifties when she came to see me. She'd had a lot of ups and downs in her weight-loss journey over the decades, and she was feeling demotivated. Halle had turned to a plant-based diet and lost about 80 pounds gradually. But then she had got busy, begun to eat processed vegan foods, and the weight came back. When we met, Halle wasn't losing weight even when she followed a strict low-fat and low-calorie diet. That's a hallmark sign of insulin resistance. She was diagnosed with type 2 diabetes and struggled to walk around the block. At 5 foot 3, she was approaching 350 pounds. She wanted to breathe easily when she walked, and secretly she dreamed of joining a local hiking club. That dream seemed impossible!

Halle was afraid to try intermittent fasting. She was so conditioned to the idea that losing weight was about losing calories that the idea of periods when she wouldn't eat felt too scary. She confessed that she used to raid the refrigerator at three in the morning because even going four hours without food was inconceivable. I encouraged her to start fasting slowly.

Halle began with time-restricted eating. First, she worked toward going 12 hours (including sleep time) without food. Over time, she changed her habits and was able to go 16 to 18 hours without eating. And the result? She lost 60 pounds just by eating her two or three meals within a 6- to 8-hour window, eliminating all snacks between meals, and cutting out all processed carbs.

Halle's biggest struggle was increasing her intake of healthy fats. She'd been told so many times that fats are bad, and even though she knew that the amount of cholesterol you eat has nothing to do with how high your cholesterol levels are, she struggled to change her mindset. But Halle persisted, and with baby steps, she made healthy changes to her habits. Although she doesn't always follow her eating and intermittent fasting plans perfectly, she has built a solid foundation. She eats a low carb, high healthy fat, mostly plant-based diet with an occasional meal that includes fish, eggs, or bacon. She's reversed her type 2 diabetes, and she no longer struggles with depression, brain fog, emotional eating, rosacea, adult acne, heartburn, morning respiratory phlegm, or joint aches. Her migraines are all but gone, and she's had a major decrease in seasonal allergy symptoms. Best of all, she has tons more energy. She now walks about five miles a day, and her longest trek with the hiking club was almost fourteen miles!

She told me, "I believe this very sustainable way of living is what has not only kept me healthy but gave me back my quality of life—it is the ultimate in self-care."

If you have trouble with any of the fasting steps, here are some extra tools—I call them fasting fluids and training wheels—to make fasting easier and more comfortable. Please use whichever of these tips your body needs—or none at all. Remember, each person's journey is different and this is *your* journey.

• FASTING FLUIDS AND TRAINING WHEELS: TWO TIPS FOR EASIER FASTING •

Trying something new can be scary; you can feel like you're taking a deep dive into unknown territory. I understand that cutting out snacks or dropping one meal a day (page 154) can feel like that. So, I want to share two tips to help make fasting easier for you. If you feel like you need support during a fast, try fasting fluids or training wheels. These liquids and easily digested foods do not provoke a significant insulin response in the body, and so they satiate any cravings you may have while allowing you to continue your fast.

Fasting fluids

Staying well hydrated while fasting helps minimize or avoid headaches and other side effects that can result as your body burns fuel and eliminates toxins. Drinking also fills your belly with liquid so you feel more satiated, and sipping can help keep your hands occupied when you are used to eating frequently.

Drink the following fluids at any time during any fast, even a "clean" fast. Clean fasting means you are consuming only water, natural salt, and magnesium *or* clear tea or coffee. You can also combine these fluids with training wheels (see below).

1 **Water:** Any temperature flat or sparkling water is the ultimate fasting fluid.

2 **Tea or coffee:** Try hot or cold tea or coffee served without sweeteners or creamers.

3 **Sugar-free pickle juice or olive brine:** Both of these fluids boost your salts and electrolytes.

Training wheels

Think of these training wheels as helping you adapt when life intrudes on your fast. Jetlag, lack of sleep, major life events, and work stress can all make it harder to complete a fast successfully. For example, if you've started a 24-hour fast but feel fatigued at 16 hours, it's better to use a training wheel than to give up the fast. You may hear some people call training wheels "dirty" fasting because consuming these things raises insulin, but I don't use this language. Many of my clients find training wheels extremely helpful when transitioning from eating many times a day to fasting successfully. Try one of these options if you need a boost as you're learning to fast.

· **Flavorings for water:** Lemon juice, lime juice, or edible essential oils can make water taste better. Try doTERRA or Young Living edible essential oils (not all essential oils are edible, so check the labels carefully). One popular combination is basil and grapefruit essential oil in carbonated water.

· **Added fat for tea or coffee:** Up to 3 teaspoons of heavy cream (use goat, sheep, or buffalo dairy if you find the A1 protein in cow's milk inflammatory), coconut milk or cream, full-fat or homogenized milk, or homemade unsweetened nut milk can make tea or coffee more satiating. Milks that are high in fat are low in sugar so they don't interfere with your fast because they don't cause an insulin surge. Avoid skim milks, which are low in fat and high in sugar; oat milk, which usually contains canola oil and is inflammatory; and store-bought nut milks, which contain additives. If you prefer, add butter or clarified butter (ghee) or medium-chain triglycerides (MCT). (Or take MCT oil on its own.)

- **Salt or cinnamon for tea or coffee:** For people who are struggling to eliminate fat from their coffee, try salt to help mask the bitterness. Salt makes coffee much more palatable for people who are used to a lot of cream and/or sugar. For people who are struggling to come off sweeteners, including stevia, use cinnamon to make the tea or coffee taste sweeter. Cinnamon is a natural anti-inflammatory too.

- **Bone broth or low-carbohydrate vegetable broth:** Broth is flavorful, and many people associate it with health. Pour broth into a bowl and eat it with a spoon to trick your mind into thinking that you are eating, to avoid drawing the attention of those around you who might interrogate you about fasting, and to model healthy eating so your family can enjoy meals together.

Once you're able to fast with ease, work on reducing and eventually eliminating these aids completely. Training wheels in particular are fuel for the body, which raises insulin and can cause people with insulin resistance to stall on their journey to wellness. In my experience, women often struggle more than men to kick the training wheels to the curb because they provide us with comfort. A cup of coffee with a few tablespoons of heavy cream doesn't seem like that big of a deal on a stressful day, right? But every time a woman agrees to cut out the cream, the weight starts to melt off, she feels better, and she finds fasting easier. Suddenly a 24-hour fast seems like a breeze and even three days of fasting become not a big deal.

In this chapter, you've begun the work of building your fasting muscle, thinking about your mindset, and making sure you know the rules of fasting. As we continue to build that fasting muscle, keep what you've learned in this chapter front of mind to root your journey in healthy and safe practices. Take the time that you need to get comfortable with these first steps and to build your confidence as you slowly change your behavior around food. By cultivating a healing mindset, setting intentional goals, and committing to cut out snacks, you're building a strong foundation for safe, healthy, and successful fasts.

Chapter 8 Takeaways

- Fasting is like a muscle. If you train yourself to fast using a step-by-step approach, you're more likely to succeed in the long run.

- Cutting out snacks can be challenging, but it is a great way to reduce inflammation, prevent weight gain, and build your fasting muscle.

- Gradually extend the time between your last meal of the day and your first meal the next morning, perhaps aiming for one 14-hour fast.

- Consistency is key. I repeat this idea throughout this book because it's very important. We'll look at why consistency is so vital, but for now work on building consistency in your early steps.

9

How to Begin and Extend Shorter Fasts

Use Fat Fasting and Drop One Meal a Day

· · · · ·

"Put yourself on a single meal a day,
now—dinner—for a few days, till you secure a
good, sound, regular, trustworthy appetite, then
take to your one and a half permanently,
and don't listen to the family any more."

MARK TWAIN

O NCE YOU'RE FEELING good about cutting out snacks and doing 14-hour fasts, it's time to consider extending your healing window and building a regular fasting practice. Remember to commit to a pace that is safe for you and that you can maintain. If you're finding it hard to manage the 14-hour fasts (or longer fasts later on), and the fasting fluids and training wheels (page 142) are not enough, try using a fat fasting approach to lengthen your healing window.

Fat fasting focuses on satiation—making sure your body feels full—which helps curb hunger cravings and allows you to start fasting fully. If you don't need the support of fat fasting, you might decide to skip this step and start to prolong your healing window by dropping one meal a day. Choose whichever approach feels right for you and your body, and know that you can change your path if needed.

Learning to Fast, Step Three: Use Fat Fasting

Fat fasting means prioritizing a diet that is high in natural fats. Dietary fat stimulates leptin production, and leptin is our primary satiation hormone—we feel full when we eat dietary fat. Fat fasting has another benefit too. Dietary fat doesn't provoke an inflammation response in the body. By eating nothing but natural fats, we avoid inciting inflammation or exacerbating it. And we avoid a problem that we haven't yet explored but which is important as we learn about feeling satiated. Leptin, a hormone that helps our bodies maintain a normal weight, can bind to inflammation rather than to our leptin receptors, and this inhibits our feeling of fullness. If we don't know that we're full, we keep on eating. And eating. When we feel full, we naturally want to stop eating. Fat fasting is designed to make you feel full by eating a few natural fats only, as often as needed. And you do it for as long as it takes for your body to stop craving food, so you can start fasting entirely. Here's how to get started.

Choose natural fats your body can tolerate

All of us have different tolerances for digesting different types and amounts of fat. If a fat food makes you feel nauseous or unpleasant, do not use it as part of your fat fasting protocol. Remember that you are what your food eats, so try to pick healthy natural fats whenever possible.

Keep your diet monotonous

Pick three or four natural high-fat foods that you enjoy and make you feel good when you consume them—say, bacon, eggs, avocados,

NATURAL FATS
Choose from these healthy fats

oils (buy organic when you can): avocado, extra-virgin olive, MCT (made from the fatty acids found in coconut oil, palm kernel oil, and certain dairy products), and macadamia nut

dairy: unprocessed cheese; full-fat cream, sour cream, and crème fraiche; ghee and butter

meat: any kind (preferably grass-fed)

poultry and eggs (preferably free-range, hormone-free, organic, and grain-fed)

fish and seafood (preferably wild, not factory farmed)

nuts: macadamia, pine, almonds, walnuts, pecans, Brazil

seeds: chia seeds

REFINED FATS
Avoid these dangerous fats whenever possible

margarine

oils: vegetable, corn, canola, grapeseed, cottonseed, safflower, sunflower, soybean, peanut

processed cheeses: slices wrapped in plastic, canned or spray cheeses, cheese sold in tubes or boxes

processed meats: bologna, hot dogs

nuts: cashews and pistachios

and olives—and make all of your meals from these foods. Don't make the mistake of too much variety. Boredom is part of what helps you to move away from frequent eating. You can even go further and make the same meal over and over again—maybe a stir-fry or an omelet. When we eat the same foods repeatedly, we lose our appetite for them and become easily sated. When I was taking exams, for example, I ate pizza every day for fourteen days until I was finished my exams. By that time, I was so sick and tired of pizza that I was no longer hungry for *anything*.

Eat any time that you're hungry

When fat fasting, you don't need to take breaks between eating, and don't try to time your meals or eat during certain windows. It's important that you focus on eating when you feel hungry because the goal of fat fasting is to gain control of your fasting muscle when you are struggling—perhaps you are new to fasting, or you are coming to fasting again after a vacation, or you are experiencing a lot of stress, or your progesterone is high—by managing satiation. On the first day of a fat fast, you might feel hungry and eat eighteen times. By day two, perhaps you feel hungry and eat nine times. By day three, many of my clients report that they feel hungry and eat only once or twice. Fasting has become easy for them, because they feel full.

Fabiana's Story

When Fabiana first came to see me, she was twenty-four years old and working the overnight shift in a factory. She ate a lot of donuts from the vending machine and was on the verge of going blind from diabetic retinopathy. She also suffered from obesity and type 2 diabetes. I recommended that she try intermittent fasting for 24 to 42 hours, three times a week, but she could not fast because she had so much inflammation in her body that any leptin she produced was binding to the inflammation and preventing her from feeling full. She was addicted to sugar and to eating.

To help break the cycle of inflammation and encourage her body to fast regularly, I asked Fabiana which two foods she'd given up that she loved when she began to fast. She said bacon and eggs. So, I told her to go home and cook 2 pounds of bacon and half a dozen eggs. I told her to eat any time she was hungry.

A week later, she had broken her habituated food cravings by eating these two natural high-fat foods over and over again. And she was able to begin fasting effectively and manage her diabetes. She has lost more than 100 pounds and come off all her insulin and hypertension medications.

My Story

I got married in Orlando, Florida, even though neither my husband nor I lived there. I went to Florida with the best intentions of eating well, but I ended up eating horribly because I was so stressed. We had planned the whole wedding in three months; our families were meeting for the first time at the wedding; and the wedding was during Christmas, so there were holiday celebrations as well. It was a lot to organize, and I felt a lot of pressure.

We spent a total of three weeks in Orlando and the experience was wonderful. But I gained quite a bit of weight. I was eating to deal with the stress, plus I kept thinking, *I should indulge! It's my wedding.* And it was the holidays. We spent a lot of time eating and celebrating.

When I got home, I was hungry all the time. I did a fat fast for two weeks to totally turn off my hunger, and that fat fast set me up to follow a consistent intermittent fasting protocol and to stick to good eating choices. I lost a lot of body fat and hit my optimal body fat percentage within two months after that fat fast because I had been patient and I allowed my body to learn how to feel full on fats.

If I know ahead of time that I'm going to be stressed—for example, I'm hosting a Christmas or Thanksgiving dinner for nineteen people—I might use fat fasting to get through the stress rather than stick to my regularly scheduled intermittent fasting period.

• FAT FASTING FAQS •

I get asked a lot of questions about fat fasting by women who are starting their fasting journey and those who are using a fat fast to get through a plateau in their journey. For example, women who are successfully managing regular intermittent fasts but want to try an extended fast can use fat fasting to help suppress their appetite during the transition. Here are some of the most commonly asked questions—and my replies.

When should I use fat fasting?

Fat fasting is versatile. I recommend it for many people who are new to fasting and having trouble making the transition from cutting out snacks to 14-hour or longer fasts. By suppressing appetite, fat fasting takes away the conditioned response to eat. For the same reason, I recommend fat fasting for people who are trying to move from a regular intermittent fasting protocol to an extended fast (see Chapter 10).

Fat fasting is helpful when the body is inflamed because it does not cause more inflammation, and it allows the body to feel full. It is a good strategy to recover from a period of poor eating or overeating, such as on a holiday or special occasion. If you've caused your body to secrete a lot of insulin because of eating constantly and consuming a lot of carbs, your body will feel heavy because it is retaining water. If you jump into a strict fast, you'll lose a ton of water and a lot of electrolytes, which causes your body extreme stress. For this reason, I always recommend that people do a fat fast to replenish electrolytes more easily and regain control of their insulin.

Can you combine fat fasting with other fasting protocols?

Yes, absolutely. You can combine fat fasting with regular fasting strategies. You allow yourself to eat when you have cravings during a fat fast, but when you're following a regular fasting protocol, you ride the hunger wave and wait until your next scheduled meal. Combining both strategies can be useful when beginning a fasting journey to learn how to manage cravings.

Can I drink fatty beverages and bone broth?

Yes, you can consume these beverages in lieu of fatty foods when fat fasting.

What are the best foods for fat fasting?

Any animal product is a great choice. Try eggs, bacon or pork belly, beef—especially a fattier cut, like ribeye. Chicken thighs and legs, as opposed to skinless chicken breast, are also a great choice. Fatty fish, like salmon, are satiating. Olive, coconut, macadamia nut oil, ghee, beef tallow, duck fat, and oil-based mayo are all going to help satiate you. Commonly I do bacon, chicken wings, and beef, along with leafy greens cooked in duck fat. If you eat plant-based foods, try cooking your leafy greens in plant oils—perhaps kale cooked in avocado oil could be one of your four foods. Avocado drizzled in olive oil is a great food to choose for a fat fast.

Should I avoid any foods while fat fasting?

Avoid dairy, nuts, and seeds, which can be inflammatory. Often people who are failing to suppress their appetite have a lot of inflammation in the body. If you are an omnivore or a carnivore, cut out all three of these food categories. If you follow a plant-based diet, cut out dairy and nuts but eat seeds so that you get enough protein. If you are a vegetarian who eats dairy, you may need to eat dairy to get enough fat.

Learning to Fast, Step Four:
Drop One Meal a Day

Once you are accustomed to living without snacks and to fat fasting, the next step is to cut out one of your three meals in the day. Most of my clients begin to fast by dropping breakfast. (This is different from *eating* one meal a day, or OMAD, which we explore a little later in the book.) This results in a 16- to 18-hour-a-day fast, depending on your mealtime. You've probably heard the phrase *16/8* or *18/6 fast* in magazines, on TV, or social media. It's also called *time-restricted eating* because by dropping one meal a day, you end up eating all your meals in a certain window of time.

Recent studies have questioned the effectiveness of time-restricted eating for losing weight.[1] And in my experience, we don't necessarily see this type of fast solving metabolic issues. But a 16/8 or 18/6 fast is great for maintaining good health or addressing mild issues, such as reducing small amounts of inflammation in the body. It is an excellent tool to help women with PCOS, type 2 diabetes, or stubborn postpartum weight build an effective fasting muscle. As in the previous three steps, dropping one meal a day gradually and safely gets you closer to a longer therapeutic fast. Here's the easiest way to drop one meal a day.

Eliminate breakfast

Breakfast is often the meal that people choose to eliminate because they don't have time to eat in the morning. Because a lot of breakfast foods in North America are laced with sugar and heavy in carbohydrates, it's a good one to drop. Think about the standard options: pancakes or cereal, French toast or waffles, toast or pastries with jam or chocolate spread. When we elect to give up eating this type of breakfast, we're helping our bodies by removing the huge sugar rush with which we usually start our day.

If you feel alarmed at the thought of skipping breakfast, you're not alone. Many of us have been told again and again that breakfast is the most important meal of the day. Once you've tried it a few times, you'll realize how easy it is. By skipping breakfast, our first meal of the day becomes lunch. In North America that generally means more healthy, whole-food options, such as green salad, meat, soup, and cooked vegetables. Remember that our healing mindset considers eating to be *rebuilding*, so select whole, healthy foods to support your body and move you more swiftly along your path to wellness.

My Story

I'd never liked breakfast, so when I first started fasting, I jumped into 16- or 18-hour fasts daily. On workdays, I did an 18-hour-a-day fast. I loved the freedom of never having to eat breakfast. My next step was to deepen my fasts by strengthening my fasting muscle. I completed three 24-hour fasts a week for a month. It was easy. Then one night I forgot to eat dinner and did my first 36-hour fast without even realizing it. This longer fast was also easy for me.

I began to experiment with extended fasts. I tried three 42-hour fasts, but my thyroid function was not very good and my adrenals were weak. And so I adjusted my fasting practice to better support my thyroid and adrenal function. As well, the cumulative stress of life and the fasts made it very difficult for me to fast on Fridays. I didn't have big plans every Friday night, but I'd usually go for dinner with friends or my husband. My therapeutic protocol became two 42-hour fasts a week, plus one 24-hour fast. I did a 42-hour fast on Mondays and Wednesdays (I ate lunch and supper on Tuesdays and Thursdays) and then I did one 24-hour fast on Fridays, starting right after dinner on Thursdays. On Saturdays and Sundays, I ate three meals each day. I did that for six months.

It's really important to keep going back to our mindset, and that's how I managed those first six months. I chose fasting as the therapy for my disease. I committed to that therapy for three times a week as I would have committed to chemo treatments. Today, I maintain a 16- or 18-hour time-restricted eating plan every day. Now that I've reached my goals, time-restricted eating helps me to maintain my health and my weight. Occasionally, I do a 24-hour fast.

My biggest challenge is that I love to snack. I don't like to cook, so I want to snack. I could eat nuts, olives, jerky, or a pack of prosciutto. With the online program, we do group challenges and every three months we do a no snacking challenge—it's everyone's struggle. Everyone's busy and snacking is just so easy. Fasting, though, has become a way of life for me—and it helps me to deal with lapses like snacking.

My husband and I were out for dinner one night at the Keg, and the people next to us had ordered everything: appetizers, salad, mains, desserts. The food just kept coming and coming. My husband said to me, "That's not just their one meal. They probably already ate today. Can we ever imagine going back to that way of eating?"

By mastering the four steps we've looked at in the last chapters— building a healing mindset, cutting out snacking, using fat fasting, and dropping one meal a day—you will build a strong foundation to move on to therapeutic fasts, the types of protocols that help you to prevent and reverse disease. Remember that if you find yourself struggling, you can always come back to these four steps. Renew your commitment to your healing goals. Rebuild your confidence by successfully cutting out snacks. Do a fat fast to curb your cravings and recalibrate your body. And then gradually drop one meal a day. In no time, you'll find yourself ready to safely and effectively tackle longer fasts.

Although we've been using a step-by-step method to learn to fast, I'd recommend that you move to a 24-hour fast three times a week as soon as you're comfortable doing so. If you've been introducing each of the four steps over the course of a month, you shouldn't experience much discomfort. The sweet spot for health for most women is a 24- to 42-hour fast, three days a week, on whichever days and times best fit into their lifestyle. We'll look at these intermittent fasts in the next chapter.

If your relationship with food has been a lifelong struggle, or even if it hasn't, a step-by-step approach can help you to incorporate therapeutic fasting into your life, even when it's difficult.

• EXPERT TIP •

Plan activities for your fasting days ahead of time so that you always have a plan of action before you get into a funk or feel hungry during your fast.

If you're always hungry at 6 p.m., for example, then hit the gym or a fitness class during that time. If you're feeling stressed about work, go for a walk instead of eating. Take an Epsom salt bath if you're feeling tired and frustrated at home, or read a book on your back porch, garden, or organize your closet instead of opening the fridge. Meet a good friend for tea or coffee. Plan a vacation for when you reach your goals.

Use this plan-ahead tip to stay on track and motivated, so you can continue to experience the benefits of fasting.

Chapter 9 Takeaways

- Use fat fasting if you're struggling with hunger. Every time you're hungry, eat a diet based on four high-fat foods until you learn to manage your cravings.

- Therapeutic fasts, which are at least 24 hours and intermittent, prevent and reduce disease most effectively. But jumping right into one of these fasts can be dangerous and ineffective. Begin by dropping one meal a day to train your fasting muscle.

- Longer fasting strategies, such as 24-, 36-, 42-, or 48-hour fasts, require a strong fasting muscle—build up to these protocols and learn how to do them effectively in the next chapter.

10

Longer Fasting Strategies
Therapeutic Fasts to Reverse and Prevent Disease

• • • • • • • • • •

"The practice, observed by many clinicians
of the old school, who advantageously fasted their diabetics
one day a week have given the cue to intermittent fasting."

DR. ELLIOTT P. JOSLIN

B Y THE TIME you get to this chapter, I'm hoping that you've spent several weeks exploring the four steps in the last two chapters. You've looked at your mindset, you've cut out snacking, perhaps you've tried fat fasting, and you've begun 16/8 or 18/6 fasts by dropping one meal a day. You've learned strategies to deal with the wave of hunger, and you're regularly able to say no when someone offers you food outside of your eating window. The shorter fasting strategies we've looked at are great to help you get used to fasting, but to cure disease and to improve health, I believe you need to explore longer fasting protocols. Therapeutic fasts have two criteria: they must be at least 24 hours, and they must be intermittent. Consistent and intermittent fasts of 24 hours or more reverse illness for women with hormonal imbalances. And in my clinical experience, longer fasts also help reverse metabolic illnesses, such as PCOS, and help with weight loss over 15 pounds.

In this chapter, we'll look more closely at how to successfully use therapeutic fasting to manage our health and cure our diseases. These are deeper, more intensive fasting experiences that can transform your body and your health, but they require commitment, consistency, and *time* to be effective. It takes ten to fifteen years to develop type 2 diabetes, which is a long time for your body to experience a way of being. The good news is that it takes less time to reverse those effects. I have seen clients reverse metabolic illness within six months of starting intermittent fasting—and I've achieved that change myself—but to do that, consistency is key. What's most important is that you **find a fasting protocol that works best for you,** so that you are consistent and successful.

Therapeutic fasting protocols vary in length, and which type of fast is right for you will depend on your current health and your healing goals. I recommend you show up for your fast like you would for any medical treatment: consistently and actively, understanding that change takes time but that you are following a tried and tested path to wellness that countless women before you have followed.

Most people find fasting three times a week to be the most sustainable and to provide the best results. However, you may start on one type of therapeutic fast and then try another as your healing goals shift. Or you might start with a 24-hour fast three times a week and slowly prolong your healing periods, to see how your body responds. Work with your doctor to determine which fast best suits your current needs. And please do review the rules of fasting (page 131) again before you make any expansive changes.

Integrating intermittent therapeutic fasts into your life can bring many benefits, and I encourage you to give them a try. Through my own experience and the experiences of thousands of clients I've worked with, I've learned a few tips to make fasting easier for you! Refer to these strategies as you progress through your fasting journey.

· TOP TEN TIPS FOR FASTING SUCCESS ·

1   Always be safe.
Our number one rule is to always be safe while fasting. If you are not feeling well, or feeling unsure of something, then stop fasting and get some help. There will always be another day to fast. Don't push yourself and get into trouble.

2   Drink more water.
Start each morning with a full 8-ounce (250 mL) glass of water. Staying hydrated keeps you feeling well.

3   Stay busy.
Choose to fast on a busy day at work. Being occupied keeps your mind off food, and gives you extra time to get your work done. A win-win situation!

4   Ride the waves.
Remember that hunger comes in waves; it's not continuous. Hunger does not keep going up and up until you eat. It peaks and then comes down. When you're hungry, think to yourself, *I'm not hungry, I'm thirsty.* Drink a glass of water or a cup of plain coffee or tea. That small action will help you move on.

5   Drink coffee or herbal tea.
Both green tea and coffee are mild appetite suppressants and contain caffeine, which helps keep your metabolic rate up. Black,

oolong, or herbal teas are also acceptable. Just remember to skip the sweeteners and creamers.

6   Shh! Don't talk about fasting.
Some people are discouraging because they do not understand the benefits of fasting. So, other than speaking to your doctor, keep the fact that you're fasting to yourself—unless you know you're going to get the support you deserve.

7   Give your body a month to adjust.
Your body needs time to get used to fasting. The first few fasts may be difficult, so be prepared. Don't get discouraged because fasting *will* get easier.

8   Fit it into your life.
Don't limit yourself socially because you're fasting. Arrange your fasting schedule to fit into your lifestyle, and adjust your fasting schedule week to week or month to month, if need be.

9   Fasting is not an excuse to eat poorly.
During nonfasting days, stick to a nutritious diet low in sugars and refined carbohydrates for best results. Remember your healing mindset: you are healing and rebuilding. Choose nourishing foods.

10 When you're finished, act like it never happened.
Fasting is not an excuse to binge eat afterward. Overeating and eating a poor diet can slow down your progress and discourage you. Remember, you're not depriving yourself when you fast, so you don't need to "reward" yourself by overeating.

We generally talk about three-fasts-a-week strategies, two-fasts-a-week strategies, and extended fasting protocols. Let's look at each of these types of fasting strategies now.

Three-Fasts-a-Week Strategies: 24- to 42-Hour Fasts

In my clinical experience, the gold standard to tackle metabolic issues for women is to do three fasts a week of 24 to 42 hours each. I've worked with over 20,000 people, and fasting three times a week seems to be the sweet spot for getting results, staying motivated, and moving forward on a path to wellness. By trying a three-fasts-a-week protocol, whether the fasts are 24, 30, 36, or 42 hours each time, women show clear results and are motivated by their success.

The reason that three times a week works well for so many people is that it builds a routine that helps to break bad eating habits. Clients know they shouldn't snack or eat unhealthy food like candy, but early in the fasting journey, it is challenging to break those ingrained bad habits. I know how hard it is because snacking is my number one challenge, and I've been fasting for years! When people don't fast frequently enough, fasting on its own doesn't break old habits around food. I regularly see women who have been dieting on and off their whole lives, and their eating habits are in a binge-and-diet cycle that has been normalized for them—depriving their bodies of nutrients and creating unhealthy relationships with food. When food is our best friend, and when we don't take breaks from eating, those old habits can be very difficult to change.

Fasting regularly, three days a week on alternate days, helps women to see results. And rather than giving up quickly, assuming that fasting is like any of the other countless diets they've tried, they are more motivated to continue changing their eating patterns because they see how fasting actually works. That said, the three-times-a-week strategy needs to be followed for six months to a year for you to see genuine, lasting results and to improve your motivation. Motivation is fleeting for many of us at the best of times, and everyone needs to see results to keep moving forward.

Pia's and Nina's Story

Identical twins from Vancouver contacted me, looking to lose weight. They were so identical that even their bloodwork was identical. They had identical body composition but very different dispositions when it came to fasting.

One twin was much more moderate. She treated fasting like a therapy: sometimes her fasts were 24 hours, sometimes they were 42, but she showed up consistently and had fantastic results. She felt confident and energetic. One year after she began fasting, she felt comfortable wearing a bathing suit with her family at the beach. She was so comfortable in her own skin that she truly enjoyed her vacation for the first time in years.

Her sister had a more extreme approach to fasting. She decided she was going to transform herself by doing a five-day fast once a month for six months—and forget about fasting all the other days of the month. After those first six months, she gave up fasting. By the end of the year, this twin hadn't lost any weight, and she hadn't gained energy. Even though she had managed longer and more extreme fasts than her sister, she hadn't maintained consistency. She had lost all motivation and felt like a failure.

If you went to the gym only once a month, you wouldn't expect to get stronger, yet this twin expected great results with longer fasts and less consistency than her sister. Remember, consistency is key—not only for losing weight and meeting your healing goals but for staying motivated.

The successful twin has maintained her fasting goals. Her sister has now adapted a moderate approach, lost weight, and feels terrific.

To successfully integrate three fasts a week, fit them in any combination that works for your schedule. You could stagger your fasts—for example, one on Monday, one on Wednesday, and one on Friday. It's great to pick days when you're busy so you are distracted, but make sure you're not so busy that you overfatigue. When I first started, I fasted Mondays, Wednesdays, and Fridays, which were my busiest workdays of the week, and I barely noticed I was fasting. I knew the weekends would be too challenging as fasting days, partly because I'd have time to look at the fridge instead of rushing from meeting to meeting! It's important, however, that you don't select a supremely busy week to begin to integrate longer fasts because then the fasting can become exhausting and dispiriting. Remember, keeping yourself motivated helps you stay consistent, and that will transform your health in the long run.

The unexpected happens to all of us, and if some weeks you can't incorporate three fasts of at least 24 hours, my advice is that you *do 16- or 18-hour fasts* to maintain results—even if those results won't be as rapid or as visible as with longer fasts.

Three 24-hour fasts per week

A 24-hour fast means dropping two meals in a row each day. Let's say you have dinner Tuesday night, then *no breakfast* and *no lunch*, and you eat dinner the next day, Wednesday. That's a 24-hour fast. But what's enjoyable about fasting is that you don't have to be exact. If you're eating 23.5 hours after your last meal, the fast will still be effective. Here's a sample fasting plan:

PLAN FOR A 24-HOUR FAST
FROM DINNER-TO-DINNER THREE TIMES A WEEK

SUNDAY	MONDAY	TUESDAY	WEDNESDAY	THURSDAY	FRIDAY	SATURDAY
FAST	FAST	FAST	FAST	FAST	FAST	FAST
Lunch	FAST	Lunch	FAST	Lunch	FAST	Lunch
Dinner	Dinner	Dinner	Dinner	Dinner	Dinner	Dinner

This 24-hour dinner-to-dinner fast works well for many of my clients, who find this timing easiest to incorporate into their lifestyle. However, some people find a 24-hour dinner-to-dinner fast very challenging—if they have an underlying thyroid condition or are dehydrated, which puts a lot of stress on their adrenal glands. They are extremely fatigued by around 4 p.m., have cravings for junk food, or experience headaches and lethargy. If this is the case, or if a 24-hour dinner-to-dinner fast conflicts with your lifestyle or work routine, try a lunch-to-lunch or breakfast-to-breakfast fast instead.

Timing might be the difference between struggle and success. In Colombia, where lunch is the focal meal of the day, many clients prefer lunch-to-lunch fasts. In other words, they eat lunch, then *no dinner* and *no breakfast*, and they eat again at lunch the next day.

PLAN FOR A 24-HOUR FAST
FROM LUNCH-TO-LUNCH THREE TIMES A WEEK

SUNDAY	MONDAY	TUESDAY	WEDNESDAY	THURSDAY	FRIDAY	SATURDAY
FAST	FAST	FAST	FAST	FAST	FAST	FAST
Lunch	Lunch	Lunch	Lunch	Lunch	Lunch	Lunch
FAST	Dinner	FAST	Dinner	FAST	Dinner	Dinner

I see clients electing to do a lunch-to-lunch fast here in North America too, especially if they have frequent cravings in the afternoon or if they have thyroid issues. A lunch-to-lunch fast can act like water wings keeping a person afloat until their thyroid and adrenal glands are strong enough to do more fasting.

Our primary stress hormone, cortisol, fluctuates throughout the day. It's highest in the morning and has a little peak around 4 p.m. before it drops so that we can sleep at night. Because of all the stressors in life—including fasting, which has a physical toll on the body—many of us lack cortisol in the afternoon, which causes us to crave junk food. You may not even like sweets, but you find you crave candy in the afternoon. That's because the sugar punches our adrenal glands into action in the afternoon, helping us produce cortisol. So, by eating lunch, you provide your body with sodium, magnesium, and vitamin B to help support the adrenal glands. When 4 p.m. rolls around, the adrenal gland has the tools it needs (nutrients) to avoid getting into that fatigued state.

Lunch-to-lunch can be better for women who have thyroid issues, either diagnosed or undiagnosed. (Many women do not know they have hypothyroidism. So many of us just accept that we are tired all the time, but in fact we have an undiagnosed thyroid issue, often caused by inflammation.) When the thyroid is deficient, it causes the adrenals to work harder, exacerbating cravings and fatigue in the afternoon. By eating lunch and supporting the adrenals, we mitigate those effects.

· HOW TO ENSURE YOUR FAST IS INTERMITTENT ·

Dropping two meals a day on its own does not make a 24-hour fast therapeutic. The fast must also be intermittent. OMAD stands for one meal a day, and it's a form of fasting where you only eat one meal a day, skipping the other two. It's not an intermittent fasting protocol; people who follow an OMAD diet do it every day. The problem with this approach is that the body adjusts to the protocol, and the metabolism slows in the same way that we see with a calorie-restriction diet. Too few calories are consumed on an OMAD diet, and our bodies adjust to the pattern. After some initial weight loss, the metabolism slows.

Women who are doing a 24-hour fast and feeding a family often find it difficult to eat one healthy meal each day. The one meal they consume may be a North American kids' diet—hot dogs or chicken fingers. What we're aiming for is a healthy, balanced approach that is also *intermittent*. If you find that eating one meal a day suits your lifestyle, then I recommend that you alternate which meal you skip so that you get the benefit of intermittent fasting without the slowing of a routine OMAD diet.

Three 30/16 fasts per week

Three 30/16 fasts per week means that you fast for 30 hours three times a week. One common way to do this is to finish lunch on one day and not eat again until supper on the following day. You skip dinner, breakfast, and lunch. For example, you might start fasting after lunch on Monday and eat again at dinner on Tuesday. And repeat on Wednesday through Thursday, and Friday through Saturday. Here's an example.

PLAN FOR A 30-HOUR FAST THREE TIMES A WEEK

SUNDAY	MONDAY	TUESDAY	WEDNESDAY	THURSDAY	FRIDAY	SATURDAY
FAST	FAST	FAST	FAST	FAST	FAST	Breakfast
Lunch	FAST	Lunch	FAST	Lunch	FAST	Lunch
FAST	Dinner	FAST	Dinner	FAST	Dinner	Dinner

Many of my clients enjoy the ease of the 30/16 schedule. The other benefit of this protocol is that you get into a deeper fat-burning fast, which generates better results and helps you learn how to fast for longer. In my clinical experience, some of the longer fasts generate the best results.

Three 36-hour fasts per week

Three 36-hour fasts per week means essentially a full day of not eating followed by a full day of eating three meals. You might have three meals on Sunday and then skip breakfast, lunch, and dinner on Monday, and repeat that fast duration two more times in the week.

PLAN FOR A 36-HOUR FAST THREE TIMES A WEEK

SUNDAY	MONDAY	TUESDAY	WEDNESDAY	THURSDAY	FRIDAY	SATURDAY
Breakfast	FAST	Breakfast	FAST	Breakfast	FAST	Breakfast
Lunch	FAST	Lunch	FAST	Lunch	FAST	Lunch
Dinner	FAST	Dinner	FAST	Dinner	FAST	Dinner

This schedule is what I call a gold standard approach for weight loss and type 2 diabetes reversal. A 36-hour fast three times a week lowers insulin levels and gets you a good 12 hours of fasting in deep fat loss. During deep fat-loss fasting, you lose about 0.5 pound of weight each time. If you're following this protocol, you'll find yourself typically losing 1.5 pounds of fat per week. Another advantage to three 36-hour fasts is the reduced cognitive load; you spend much less time keeping track of schedules or thinking about eating. My clients deeply enjoy their meals, see excellent fasting results, and enjoy the freedom of not having to stop their days to eat until it's time to break their fast.

Three 42-hour fasts per week

Three 42-hour fasts per week is more or less the same as three 36-hour fasts a week, *except* you don't eat breakfast on the days you break your fast. So, you might have supper on Sunday, fast all day Monday, and skip breakfast on Tuesday. Then you plan a healthy and nutritious lunch on Tuesday, reintroducing your body to food after the long break. And repeat that cycle through the week.

PLAN FOR A 42-HOUR FAST THREE TIMES A WEEK

SUNDAY	MONDAY	TUESDAY	WEDNESDAY	THURSDAY	FRIDAY	SATURDAY
FAST	FAST	FAST	FAST	FAST	FAST	FAST
Lunch	FAST	Lunch	FAST	Lunch	FAST	Lunch
Dinner	FAST	Dinner	FAST	Dinner	FAST	Dinner

This protocol can be very effective at avoiding the dawn effect (see below) because with 42-hour fasts most people do not eat until lunchtime. Early in the morning, we naturally experience a rise in blood glucose as our body prepares for the day. Many women who are in a rush in the morning will eat something quick, like sugary cereal. They are introducing a lot of sugar after a long period without food, and added to the dawn effect, it makes them feel terrible. Taking time to plan a healthy meal post-fast is crucial, but a 42-hour fast can also help.

· THE DAWN EFFECT ·

The dawn effect, also called the dawn phenomenon, is created by the circadian rhythm. In the morning, hormone triggers wake us up. Our body secretes higher levels of noradrenaline and cortisol to give us energy for the coming day. It also secretes glucagon, which moves glucose from storage into the blood so it's available as fuel when we become active. This normal hormonal surge tells the liver to push out any excess sugar that it hasn't converted to fat, giving the body a chance to burn it off. Most people don't notice this bump in their blood glucose levels, but the spike can be very noticeable for people with type 2 diabetes. For this reason, I really encourage type 2 diabetics to *not* eat in the morning.

When blood sugar levels go up, the pancreas produces insulin in response. If you fast in the morning, you get to eliminate that sugar. But if you eat in the morning, you add more insulin to your system, adding more fuel to a fire that you're trying to put out.

The dawn effect is the hardest thing to change if you have type 2 diabetes. As you fast, you will see your bloodwork improve, especially your hemoglobin, but your morning blood sugar will still be high. It's the last thing to get better. This is why we sometimes recommend that type 2 diabetics don't check their bloodwork in the morning, unless they are taking insulin and need to balance that. By not checking your blood levels, you reduce stress and proceed with a suitable fasting protocol; however, all of this work has to be done with *medical support*.

Plan your three-times-a-week fast

Now that we've looked at three-times-a-week fasting strategies, try sketching out a plan for three fasts you intend to practice this week. Dinner isn't the focal meal for everyone, so adapt your fasting periods to end with whichever meal of the day is most important for you or best fits your schedule. Remember, it's beneficial to vary your daily eating pattern.

	M	T	W	T	F	SAT	SUN
BREAKFAST							
LUNCH							
DINNER							

Two-Fasts-a-Week Strategies: 48-, 66-, and 72-Hour Fasts

Fasting three times a week can be challenging to manage while running a household, preparing meals, and juggling work, and so many women prefer two fasts a week instead. In my home, this strategy works well. I do most of the cooking, and when I fast twice a week for 48 hours, I miss only two meals with my husband while still getting all the benefits of a longer fast. Two 48-hour fasts don't equate to the same number of hours as three 42-hour fasts, but the deeper fast and the deeper fat burning of a 48-hour fast can be easier to put into practice and very motivating as results are seen rapidly.

There are no negative repercussions to trying these longer fasts and seeing if they work for your body and your lifestyle, but do remember the rules of fasting (page 131), which are absolutely key. Be aware that these longer fasts—generally 36 hours or more—can disturb your sleep at first. Your body will adapt, but magnesium supplements can make a difference (see Chapter 11). If you're going to do a 66-hour or even a 72-hour fast, don't expect to fit one (or two) into your life every single week.

Two 48-hour fasts per week

Two 48-hour fasts per week means eating supper on Sunday and then fasting all day on Monday, skipping breakfast and lunch on Tuesday, and breaking your fast with dinner on Tuesday evening. Then you'd eat all three meals on Wednesday. You'd fast all day Thursday, and resume eating on Friday at suppertime.

PLAN FOR A 48-HOUR FAST TWICE A WEEK

SUNDAY	MONDAY	TUESDAY	WEDNESDAY	THURSDAY	FRIDAY	SATURDAY
FAST	FAST	FAST	FAST	FAST	FAST	FAST
Lunch	FAST	FAST	Lunch	FAST	FAST	Lunch
Dinner	FAST	Dinner	Dinner	FAST	Dinner	Dinner

Two 66-hour fasts per week

Two 66-hour fasts per week means that after dinner on Sunday, for example, you fast all day Monday and Tuesday, and you break your fast with lunch on Wednesday. You could do a second 66-hour fast, starting after supper on Wednesday. So, you fast all day Thursday and Friday, and resume eating at lunchtime on Saturday. You can also combine one 66-hour fast with another shorter fast each week, perhaps a 24-hour or a 42-hour fast.

PLAN FOR A 66-HOUR FAST TWICE A WEEK

SUNDAY	MONDAY	TUESDAY	WEDNESDAY	THURSDAY	FRIDAY	SATURDAY
FAST	FAST	FAST	FAST	FAST	FAST	FAST
Lunch	FAST	FAST	Lunch	FAST	FAST	Lunch
Dinner	FAST	FAST	Dinner	FAST	FAST	Dinner

Women and men respond differently to hunger and to fasting. When men start fasting, the hormone that signals hunger, ghrelin, drops quite a lot in the first 24 hours and then stabilizes. As a result, they get hunger spikes as ghrelin naturally cycles up and down throughout the day. However, when women start fasting, ghrelin comes down and stays down. This means that once a woman is into a fast, if she stays in the fast, she doesn't get hungry in the same way that a man does. For some women, a 66-hour protocol can therefore be very successful. This fast is a very good way to reduce inflammation, reduce insulin resistance, and fit fasting into your lifestyle.

One 72-hour fast plus one shorter fast per week

A 72-hour fast means you might fast after Sunday dinner and all day Monday and Tuesday, breaking your fast with supper on Wednesday. My clients who use this protocol do a 72-hour fast once a week with an additional 24-hour fast at the end of their week, on a Friday, say.

PLAN FOR A 72-HOUR FAST PLUS A 24-HOUR FAST

SUNDAY	MONDAY	TUESDAY	WEDNESDAY	THURSDAY	FRIDAY	SATURDAY
FAST	FAST	FAST	FAST	FAST	FAST	FAST
Lunch	FAST	FAST	FAST	Lunch	FAST	Lunch
Dinner	FAST	FAST	Dinner	Dinner	Dinner	Dinner

Some women like this fasting protocol because they find it easier than fasting on alternate days due to hunger pangs. Our hunger hormone, ghrelin, drops around the 36-hour mark, so as these women get to the end of their 36-hour fast, their appetite decreases and the fast feels easy. For this reason, the 72-hour fast can be very successful because they're not dealing with the aggravation of feeling hunger, they fear fasting less, and they are able to be more consistent.

The second half of the week, when the 72-hour fast is over, can be very challenging for some women. They find it tempting to lapse into old eating habits during the four days they are not fasting. Throwing in a 24-hour fast later in the week can help manage their new lifestyle.

Extended Fasting Protocols

While I think consistency with shorter or longer intermittent fasting is what gets people the bulk of their results, there is a time and a place for multiday fasts. I consider any fast beyond three days to be an extended fast, but within the fasting community an extended fast is usually five to seven days. When I was traveling a lot for work and eating poorly on the road, I would do an extended fast four times a year to reset my body and to help maintain my good health. I thought of these five-to-seven-day fasts for disease prevention, anti-aging, and hormonal reset like seasonal cleanings of my body. I would clean my house and my body at the same time: I'd use the time I was fasting to scrub my entire home from top to bottom. This approach had two benefits for me: I was so busy cleaning my house that I didn't think about food or being hungry, and I pictured overhauling my body and my home all at once, which kept me motivated and gave me a great sense of satisfaction.

Extended fasting protocols require support, and I like to monitor my clients when they do one. What I have found is **a regular intermittent fasting protocol with occasional extended fasts of five to seven days is most successful**. The longest I've allowed a patient to fast for is twenty-one days. I imagine you're wondering how they stayed hydrated and weren't starving. There are so many myths about intermittent fasting and a lot of fearmongering around starvation and dehydration. If you haven't already, I recommend you review the earlier section on common myths around women and fasting (page 21) to reassure yourself before we move forward. Extended fasts are useful for breaking through a stubborn fasting plateau (which we'll look at later). Consider trying five or seven days once a year for the benefits of autophagy.

Intermittent and extended fasting induces autophagy

The term *autophagy* refers to a physiological phenomenon in the body. The word itself comes from the Greek: *auto* means *self* and *phagy* means *to eat*, so the word translates to "eat oneself." In fact, autophagy is the body's mechanism for turning all the old and broken-down "machinery" into new and useful parts.

Before 2016 when Japanese cell biologist Yoshinori Ohsumi won a Nobel Prize for his lab work on autophagy, no one knew much about how the body destroyed and recycled its cellular components. His work garnered international attention because it explained how our body hunts down old and inactive proteins and puts them back together into new proteins and cells, like a recycling program. You take the old and you turn it into new. And you can turn it on or off by fasting.

Autophagy has been described as the body's way of cleaning out damaged cells in order to regenerate newer, healthier cells. What's remarkable is that the new cells do not have to be in the same part of the body as the old ones. What I see in clients is that they prevent disease, heal their bodies, *and* reduce the signs and symptoms of aging when their fasting induces autophagy. The results can be striking. I once failed to recognize one of my patients because her physical appearance had changed so much. She looked so much more youthful because she had induced autophagy in her body through fasting.

Ella's Story

Ella was 5 foot 5 inches and in her late sixties. Through an intermittent fasting protocol of two 48-hour fasts per week, she had recently lost 165 pounds. When she came to see me, she was delighted but surprised: "I thought I would have drapes of loose skin, but I have none."

I explained that when we gain weight, our body has to support that fat. Just like when we have a child, we have to support that child. Our body produces connective tissue to support that fat. When we start to lose fat and our cells shrink, we still have the excess connective tissue, but that connective tissue is no longer serving a function. Autophagy identifies the old cells and redistributes the connective tissue—this excess loose skin—repurposing it in other parts of the body. Ella had no draping loose skin because of the beautiful benefits of autophagy. I've also noticed women lose their C-sections scars, again because they have induced autophagy.

Unfortunately, if a woman already has loose skin from losing weight on another type of diet, I haven't seen skin reduction when they start to fast. It seems that it's generally best to lose the weight at the same time as losing the skin. A lot of clinical research on autophagy is happening at the moment, and I expect more studies will reveal why this is.

Ella graduated from our program feeling strong, healthy, and ready to maintain her transformed body. She moved into time-restricted eating with the occasional 24-hour fast to keep herself feeling her best.

There are three ways to induce autophagy in the body. The first is through intense exercise. The second is through the keto diet, a very low carbohydrate diet that forces the body to switch from glucose burning to fat burning. The bulk of food on a keto diet is natural fats or proteins, and the body becomes very efficient at burning fat for energy, a process known as ketosis. Both of these ways are hard to sustain: it's difficult to train intensively enough to maintain autophagy, and the keto diet is based on stringent restrictions that can be limiting and tough to stick to.

The third way to induce autophagy is by fasting. Researchers don't know exactly when autophagy starts to happen in the body, but for the average adult female on a whole-food diet, autophagy seems to occur sometime after 24 hours of fasting. When women fast for 30 hours and beyond, autophagy is induced. As you reverse metabolic disease, you can enter this state of autophagy through maintenance fasts, which are the shorter fasts, but very few studies have measured this. In my experience, when autophagy begins varies from woman to woman—and is impacted by stress, sleep, and travel. So, it's worth experimenting, with the support of a medical professional, to see if autophagy is happening in your body and what its effects are.

• THE PROCESS OF AN EXTENDED FAST •

- For the first hours of a fast, we are burning off the fuel from our last meal and the day before.

- Your body then starts to deplete its glycogen stores, and this takes up the first 24 hours of your fast.

- As you move into the second day, your body relies on fat for fuel. This can be very challenging. You can get stuck between a rock and a hard place: your insulin starts to block your fat stores, which can make you feel energy-depleted. Insulin, as you remember, is a fat-trapping hormone, so if you have a lot of insulin circulating in your blood, it will trap the fat. You need to suppress the insulin in your body to access the fat stores, so you struggle with burning body fat if your insulin levels are high. You want to take it easy on day 2, and use plenty of the fasting training wheels to provide your body with temporary support.

- Once your insulin levels start to come down (and they will come down), you start to feel well again. It might take 24 hours for insulin to be low enough that you release enough fat fuel for the fast to become easier. Remember, hydration is key.

- After 48 hours, the fast should get significantly easier so long as you're properly hydrated.

- On day three, you should start to feel energized and really good, with lots of mental clarity and next to no appetite. The desire to eat vanishes, even if people around you are eating. It's usually smooth sailing after the third day. The more you fast, the less of an issue it is. On a second or third extended fast, you have better tools and the learning curve is covered as your body gets used to the journey.

Women should expect different results than men

Women should expect to lose 0.5 pound of body fat per fasting day. If you do three fasts a week, that means 1.5 pounds a week of body fat loss.

Initially, you may appear to be losing a lot of weight, but it's water weight. Remember that insulin retains water, and as you shed it during your fasting journey, it can look like you're losing a lot of weight. Women lose a lot of water at the start of their fasting journey but not a lot of fat. As fasting begins to heal the hormonal imbalances that keep insulin high, the fat loss starts to happen more rapidly.

Men often lose a pound a day when they begin to fast, and then several weeks later, they level out to lose 0.5 pound of fat per fasting day. After four to six weeks of consistent intermittent fasting, women start to lose fat at the same rate as men—0.5 pound of fat per fasting day.

Don't lose hope during that middle period when you've lost a lot of water weight but aren't shedding fat, particularly if you are fasting alongside men. My advice is to hang in there, to keep going, and to trust the process. Be consistent and the results will come.

· TOP TIPS FOR EXTENDED FASTING ·

1 Hydrate consistently, especially during the first 48 hours.

2 Begin your fast when you are feeling calm and life isn't too stressful. If you fast during stressful times, the stress itself creates an insulin response, which makes burning fat more challenging and makes you feel awful physically.

3 Make sure to use those training wheels! If you fast during a busy time, you may not remember to hydrate well. Often if clients are too busy, they break the fast with quick and easy foods that are very unhealthy. A little planning at the start of a longer fast will make it much easier and more successful overall.

4 When you fast, you produce a lot of noradrenaline, which is a form of adrenaline, and many people experience insomnia as a result. If I had a busy week at work with huge projects, I would not also do an extended fast, because of the interruption to sleep. You want to find a balance between being busy enough to be distracted from thinking about eating and being too busy where sleep disruptions will be a big problem. (I explore this

further in the next chapter.) It's worth noting that noradrenaline is so high during an extended fast that there's not much you can do to reduce the insomnia. During shorter fasts, you can use oral magnesium supplements to counteract the effects of noradrenaline.

The first time I did a seven-day fast, I thought I had enough fuel to get through. But on day two and day three, I thought I was going to die. I used training wheels to help me through those feelings and made sure to hydrate and rest. When I awoke on the fourth day, my fuel tank was full because my body was finally burning fat. I felt like a whole new person. I ended up doing an eleven-day fast. I drank water, tea, and the occasional cup of broth when I needed it.

Therapeutic fasting protocols, whether two or three days a week or multiday extended fasts, combined with a low carbohydrate, high healthy fat diet are the key to reversing disease and maintaining good health. We've looked at ways to fit these fasts into your lifestyle and to induce autophagy so that you lose weight, manage hormonal imbalances, and slow the aging process.

Even if you take a step-by-step approach to fasting, you may still encounter moments when you feel unwell or when your body is changing in ways you haven't anticipated. In the next chapter, I'll walk you through some of the side effects you may experience when you fast, along with a few troubleshooting tips to make the journey easier.

Chapter 10 Takeaways

- Longer fasting protocols are therapeutic: these fasts lead to greater, more sustained weight loss and better overall health.

- Consistency is crucial. It's better to do regular, repeated shorter fasts than to do intense long fasts sporadically.

- One meal a day (OMAD) is not an intermittent fasting protocol. While skipping the same two meals a day can be convenient, your body adapts to the new eating routine and your metabolism slows.

- During longer fasts, the body dumps water weight before it begins to burn fat. Proper hydration is key.

- After 24 to 30 hours of fasting, autophagy is induced, which means the body repairs itself by recycling old broken cells into new healthy ones. We are only beginning to understand autophagy, and I anticipate new research breakthroughs over the next few years.

- I recommend an extended fast one to four times a year to detoxify your body and reset your hormones. Consult your doctor first and use medical support.

11

Tips and Tricks for Troubleshooting Fasts

• • • • •

"A fast is better than a bad meal."

IRISH PROVERB

WHETHER YOU'RE FOLLOWING shorter or longer protocols, fasting can bring great health benefits. If you're maintaining a low carbohydrate, high healthy fat diet, fasting regularly and intermittently, and avoiding foods or fluids that elicit a strong insulin response in the body, you're well on your way.

But as you would beginning an exercise program or learning any new skill, you may encounter some bumps along the road. As you develop a new relationship with food, and your body adjusts to new ways of healing and rebuilding, you may wonder if what you're feeling is "normal," or if you should be worried and seek medical advice.

As the body heals, you may find that your metabolism changes. I like to say that I've been nineteen different versions of myself. What this means, for example, is that early in my fasting journey, salt was not helpful for me. But as my body changed in response to fasting, I've had to reevaluate. Sometimes I now add salt to support my fasts or reduce unwanted side effects. Similarly, my tolerance for carbs, fats, and every other food, especially protein, has also changed along my nineteen different metabolic journeys. There have been several times throughout my life when I've been unable to fast—due to brain fog or sugar cravings—as my body has changed. What I recommend is that you anticipate that your metabolic needs will change as you heal.

In this chapter, I'll highlight some of the most common side effects you might encounter and offer easy solutions to resolve or mitigate their symptoms. I'll share with you some of the other questions I'm asked most frequently and the advice I share to motivate, reassure, and ensure success for my clients.

Common Side Effects: Symptoms and Solutions

My clients and I have encountered many of the same positive and negative side effects on our fasting journeys, and I'm here to reassure you that most unpleasant side effects are expected, short-lived, and easy to remedy. In most cases, they are not a reason to stop fasting. They are your body dumping water, sugar, or toxins, and they are stepping stones to better health.

Constipation

Bowel movements do slow down when we fast because when we don't eat, waste doesn't pass through. Sometimes clients think they're constipated because they haven't had a bowel movement. But there's a difference between not having any waste to pass and being constipated. If you have the urge to go but you can't, you're constipated. My best advice is to be patient. However, if you are experiencing discomfort or pain, try some physical movement. Exercise can help you feel good, boost your energy levels when you're fasting, and stimulate your bowels. Be sure to drink 1 cup of water for every tea or coffee too.

Recommended: If exercise and water don't get your bowels moving, try taking 400 milligrams of magnesium citrate per day. It's universally recommended to help with constipation, whether you are fasting or not. And if all else fails, try adding 1 to 2 tablespoons of MCT oil or coconut oil to your coffee or taking it straight. (This oil is also a training wheel, see page 143.) These oils are rapidly digested, and the body is usually quick to eliminate them.

Dehydration

Hydration is critical throughout any fast, and especially during the first 48 hours. That's when the body experiences the largest drop in insulin and signals the kidneys to release water. For every gram of glycogen stored, our body stores 4 grams of water. So, as we move into our fast and burn up those glycogen stores, the body gets rid of excess water by dumping it out through urination and bowel movements. Any time we lose water, we lose electrolytes, especially sodium and magnesium. In the first 48 hours of the fast, we can become electrolyte deficient, which causes brain fog, nausea, and several unwanted side effects. If you're not replenishing water through those 48 hours, you can cause a stress response, which will prevent weight loss and make you feel awful.

Dehydration is very common and often misdiagnosed. A patient of mine went on a long flight and became dehydrated, and a doctor suggested she needed to go on dialysis to save her kidneys. She came to our clinic, and it was apparent that she was dehydrated. She drank water and rehydrated and never needed the dialysis.

TROUBLESHOOTING DEHYDRATION CAUSED BY LOW ELECTROLYTES

Electrolytes are a form of a nutrient, and they are involved in every aspect of the body from how your heart pumps to how you sneeze! They are important in the maintenance of many bodily systems, and we need to make sure that we get enough of them when we are fasting and eating. On a longer fast, in the first two to three days, you'll need pickle juice, Epsom salt baths, and water so that you replenish those electrolytes. Make sure you drink when you're thirsty, and don't drink too much if you're not feeling thirsty at all. Your kidneys are like a flower: if you under-water, they don't function well; if you over-water, they don't function well. You can potentially drown from drinking too much water, so make sure you balance your hydration with salts. True hydration isn't only about replenishing liquid but also about replenishing electrolytes; sodium and magnesium are key.

If you're not replenishing sodium in the way the body antici-pates during a fast, you'll feel tired and eventually the body will become alarmed and start to shed magnesium. You also lose mag-nesium through urination and bowel movements, so watching your magnesium level is important. Low magnesium causes the body to eliminate phosphorus, calcium, and potassium too. However, if you *replenish sodium and maybe a little magnesium*, then you keep the other electrolytes in the body in balance. I like to explain it to clients like this: a magnesium supplement when fasting is akin to taking a prenatal vitamin while pregnant. The prenatal vitamin is an insurance policy that you're getting all the right nutrients. In the same way, if you focus on getting enough sodium and magnesium, you don't need to worry about the other electrolytes. Remember, hydration is *not* just water; it's water, sodium, and magnesium.

Recommended: Drink 8 to 16 ounces of water and a bit of salt (add a little to water or take it on its own), or a cup of broth or pickle juice every two to four hours a day on fasting days. Take a magne-sium supplement (see below), and avoid electrolyte drinks, which are loaded with sugar. The daily recommended dosage of magne-sium by Health Canada is 400 milligrams. But research shows that people with type 2 diabetes and metabolic syndrome benefit from taking 2,000 to 2,400 milligrams of magnesium.[1] Most individuals can't tolerate this much a day, and it's very expensive. So, I recom-mend that women combine transdermal magnesium (magnesium through the skin), magnesium oil (both of which absorb differently and do not impact the bowel), and a magnesium supplement, whether they are fasting or not.

• EXPERT TIP •

Magnesium is involved in millions of bodily functions. It helps balance our nervous system. It promotes relaxation. It helps maintain good mood and helps with sleep. It reduces symptoms of anxiety and depression. It's really important for preventing muscle cramps, or lactic acid buildup.

Most women are deficient in magnesium, and insulin resistance further depletes magnesium. People who are insulin resistant need twice as much magnesium as other people. Yet many doctors do not test these levels well. They order a magnesium serum blood test, which doesn't measure how much magnesium is in our tissues, only what is circulating in our blood. But to keep the blood levels high, the body sheds magnesium from our tissues! If you want to know whether your tissue levels are good, do a magnesium red blood cell (RBC) test.

I recommend magnesium supplements for all women, whether they are fasting or not. Magnesium citrate is a great source if you're prone to constipation. Magnesium bis-glycinate is a good alternative if you're not. Magnesium malate is excellent if you're feeling chronic fatigue. And magnesium l-threonate is the only type to cross the blood-brain barrier and has a positive impact on our mood and cognitive function; it's a good option if you don't want to be grouchy as your body acclimates to burning body fat.

Combine magnesium supplements with transdermal magnesium and magnesium oil to be sure your body absorbs this mineral. But remember to keep your sodium levels up so your body doesn't shed so much magnesium. If you're not fully absorbing magnesium, consider another way to get this crucial electrolyte in your system—foot soaks are my favorite!

One patient of mine refused to use transdermal magnesium. The prescription-grade magnesium I gave her didn't bring up her levels, which were drastically low. She was very overweight, grumpy, worried, depressed, and suffered from insomnia. In the end, she tried a foot soak, and this dramatically improved her magnesium levels. She found herself to be less grumpy, calmer, sleeping better, managing her weight and fasting well, and her magnesium levels became normal.

Diarrhea

Loose stools or bowel urgency are not uncommon when people start to fast, but generally only when a fast lasts for more than 24 hours. Sometimes it's because insulin is low: if insulin drops a lot, our kidneys signal the body to release water, which is sometimes excreted through the stool. This diarrhea can be confusing: you haven't eaten, so you don't understand why you're losing stool. Diarrhea can lead to electrolyte loss, which contributes to dehydration, fatigue, headaches, and generally feeling unwell.

Sometimes when we break our fast, we will have diarrhea. This side effect is because the body is confused by the new fasting protocol, and so it conserves digestive juices. When we break our fast, digestive enzymes aren't available to digest the food. The result is undigested food in the stool and very loose stool. Doing shorter fasts first helps to train our body before we do longer fasts, so that it doesn't conserve digestive juices but produces them normally. It usually takes two weeks for the body to adjust to the new fasting schedule and for normal digestion to resume when people have their break-fast meal. Extending your regular fasting schedule can cause these stool side effects again as your body adapts. If you stick to a consistent fasting plan, the side effects will fade within two to four weeks.

TROUBLESHOOTING DIARRHEA CAUSED BY LOW INSULIN OR LACK OF DIGESTIVE JUICES

Gas pain, bloating, and in rare cases vomiting can be signs that the body is not producing enough digestive juices. Certain foods are difficult for the digestive system to process, and to reduce these gastric symptoms when breaking fast, we suggest people avoid high fiber, high fat foods and foods that cause inflammation, like dairy. These foods can be difficult for the digestive system to process:

- alcohol

- dairy products (look for casein A1 and casein A2 if you must consume dairy)

- eggs

- nut butters

- nuts

- raw vegetables

- red meat

If you aren't having issues, then don't change your diet. If you've been fasting for a long time, your body can tolerate many of these foods. But if you are having side effects, change your break-fast foods. And it's never a good idea to consume alcoholic beverages on an empty stomach.

Recommended: Break your fast with cooked vegetables, soups, fish, or poultry, which are easy on the digestive system. If you must eat red meat, choose high-quality ground meat and eat less than usual (for example, 8 ounces rather than 12). If you find bone broth is moving through you quickly because it's too greasy, try another brand or make your own.

Fatigue

Many women experience tiredness a lot of the time, even when they are not fasting. This fatigue is often because of insulin resistance in the body. When our cells need energy, insulin resistance stops our bodies from being able to access the glucose in our blood. And we feel tired. Another common cause of fatigue for women is hypothyroidism that is undiagnosed or diagnosed and poorly managed.

A third cause of fatigue is low sodium. Insulin is a water-retaining hormone, and so when our insulin levels are high, our body retains more water. As we begin to fast and our insulin levels come down, our kidneys need to offload that water. When women fast, insulin levels drop rapidly. Women initially experience increased urination and lose electrolytes. Losing electrolytes results in low sodium levels—and one side effect is fatigue. This is different from the fatigue caused by insulin resistance or hypothyroidism, but it feels the same.

Each of these forms of fatigue calls for a different solution.

TROUBLESHOOTING FATIGUE CAUSED BY LOW SODIUM

Headaches, dizziness, mental fog, and lethargy that accompany your fatigue are signs of lower salt levels. Drink olive brine or pickle juice, or place salt crystals under your tongue to alleviate these side effects.

The body assesses its sodium levels throughout the day, so be careful not to take too much salt at once—*it can make you feel worse*. You may experience heart palpitations along with bloating and discomfort.

If you have a lot of insulin resistance, you won't experience fatigue because of low sodium when you start fasting because insulin causes salt to be retained in the body. However, once you've purged that excess insulin—maybe a few weeks into a fasting schedule—you may suddenly experience these side effects of low sodium. For example, women with type 2 diabetes may not tolerate salt when they begin fasting but find they need it later on.

Recommended: Take a pinch of salt every two to three hours a day on fasting days. (See also the section on dehydration.)

· EXPERT TIP ·

It's best to supplement with sodium throughout the day instead of waiting until you become unwell to do so. Have a pinch of salt in the morning, add salt to your coffee, and/or drink a cup of bone broth at lunchtime. Many teas and all coffees are diuretics, so they increase urinary output. Make sure you're having one glass of water for every cup of tea or coffee, and *add that salt*! Remember the salt cuts down on the bitterness of the coffee too!

TROUBLESHOOTING FATIGUE CAUSED BY HYPOTHYROIDISM AND INSULIN RESISTANCE

Fatigue caused by hypothyroidism and insulin resistance isn't connected to fasting but to the illnesses themselves. While you may feel fatigue due to IR or your thyroid, my clients find that as they progress through their healing journey, this type of fatigue goes away. This type of fatigue isn't something we can troubleshoot except by continuing with our fasting journey and healing.

A potential side effect of fasting if you do have thyroid issues is that you may need to adjust your medication as you shift from hypothyroidism to hyperthyroidism. This happens because you are healing and decreasing cellular inflammation and lowering insulin levels. The thyroid hormone can then get into cells, which it hasn't been able to do before due to inflammation. Depending on how much thyroid medication you are using, you may need to adjust or come off your medication, and this has to be done with your health-care provider.

Hashimoto's thyroiditis, which is an autoimmune disorder, destroys the thyroid gland. If your thyroid has been completely destroyed, you will always need to take thyroid medication. If you haven't had too much thyroid gland damage, you may be able to reduce your medication significantly.

If you are having issues with your thyroid and medication, I recommend that you stop fasting until your thyroid has stabilized and you have had your bloodwork done, then resume fasting again when your medication is adjusted correctly.

Gout

Gout is a metabolic disease caused by high levels of uric acid that causes painful inflammation to the joints. If you have a history of gout, it can flare up when you start to fast. As your insulin levels drop and the kidneys signal the release of excess water, your sodium levels can fall, which can result in gout.

I would never start someone with a history of gout on an extended fast. For someone whose uric acid levels are high and who has a history of gout, I would recommend they start fasting very slowly. To mitigate the effects of gout as much as possible, do not shy away from taking supplements—and consult your doctor if symptoms intensify.

Recommended: Make sure that you're getting enough salt while fasting. I also recommend adding lime juice to your water, up to 3 tablespoons throughout the day. Lime juice (not lemon juice) dissolves the uric acid associated with gout. Cherry root extract, which does not break your fast, is another great way to reduce symptoms of gout. Follow the dosage recommended on the package.

Hair loss

When body composition changes, some people suffer from head hair loss. This side effect is common during fasting, and it's due not only to the rapid change in body composition but also to the hormonal fluctuations during weight loss. Note that this hair loss is not the same as alopecia, which is a genetic condition that causes hair loss, or thyroid-related hair loss, although the symptom is the same. If you experience hair loss, check in with your doctor.

Once body composition stabilizes, the hair loss stops, across all age groups and sexes. For example, once your body has settled into losing 1 pound a week instead of, say, 5 pounds a week at the start of your fasting journey, hair loss stops. Normal hair growth then resumes.

Recommended: Be patient and wait out the hair loss. As with most fasting side effects, hair loss usually subsides within four to six weeks. For women who find waiting for hair loss to stop too challenging, or if it hasn't subsided, I recommend adding 30 grams of protein to your meals on eating days. The added protein slows weight loss, but it also completely stops hair loss for most people. You can also fast less—use a 24-hour fast instead of a 36-hour fast, for example.

Insomnia

Many women have experienced disturbed sleep, and one of the benefits of intermittent fasting is that it is associated with better sleep in the long run. However, in the short term, when starting to fast or increasing the length of your regular fasts, insomnia—the inability to get enough sleep, or high-quality sleep, despite having plenty of opportunity—is one of the most common side effects. The best thing to do is be consistent with your fasts and wait out the insomnia.

Fasting can trigger a spike in cortisol and an increase in nor-adrenaline, which provides a lot of energy. This surge of energy is great during the daytime but can be very challenging when it's time to sleep. Fasting also increases your metabolic rate and causes your insulin levels to drop—both of which are good. However, irregular levels of insulin can, for a while, increase the production of orexin, a neuropeptide that can increase energy and reduce sleep.

Recommended: Be patient, practice good sleep hygiene, choose a less busy period work to fast, and wait out the insomnia, typically up to two weeks. If the insomnia is very challenging, draw a hot bath, add 2 cups of Epsom salts, and soak for thirty minutes about an hour before bed, or take 400 milligrams of magnesium thirty minutes before bed. Many of my clients do a combination of both a bath and the magnesium supplement, either at the same time or alternating them, and find that it calms their nervous system and helps them sleep.

Keto breath

Keto breath is very bad breath. No one may want to kiss you or be around you, and you may be self-conscious, but it does mean that you're burning body fat. It's a great thing: it means the fast is working! When there is not enough glucose to supply the body's fuel needs, you're primarily fueling off fatty acids called ketone bodies. Free fatty acids are also liberated. One of these ketone bodies is acetone, which we exhale because it doesn't serve any physiological purpose in the body. The chemical taste associated with keto breath is that acetone, and it's often accompanied by a white film on the tongue.

In rare cases, keto breath lasts for a long time, but for most people it passes within a month or two as weight loss starts to slow.

Recommended: Maintain good dental hygiene by brushing, including your tongue, and flossing regularly and drink more water. You can also try oil pulling: scoop or pour a tablespoon of edible oil (perhaps coconut or avocado oil) into your mouth, let it melt, and swish it around for twenty minutes (while in the shower or emptying the dishwasher, for example) without swallowing it. The fat is antimicrobial, and by swishing it around, you're deep-cleaning your mouth. Don't spit it down the drain because it will solidify, clogging the pipes. I suggest you spit it into a cup, let it harden, and then throw it away. Afterward, rinse your mouth with salt water and brush your teeth. If you're worried about persistent keto breath, however, seek out medical attention.

Muscle cramps

Muscle cramps are usually harmless, but they can be painful. When fasting, you may occasionally experience spasms or sharp pains in your legs or joints or an overall aching feeling. These cramps and aches are often a side effect of low magnesium caused by dehydration. When we fast, our insulin levels drop and we start to rapidly excrete excess water. When we dump that water, we lose sodium. When our sodium levels get too low, our body sheds magnesium, which causes the muscle cramps.

TROUBLESHOOTING MUSCLE CRAMPS
CAUSED BY LOW MAGNESIUM

The number one recommendation is soaking in a warm bath with Epsom salts; the magnesium in the salts is absorbed through your skin. If you don't want to go this route, I recommend buying magnesium oil or gel to rub onto your feet about thirty minutes before a shower, or even to leave it on throughout the night. You do not need to wash it off, but it can leave a white filmy residue on your skin.

You can make your own magnesium oil at home. Use equal parts Epsom salts and distilled water. Dissolve the Epsom salts in boiling distilled water. And as my husband, an organic chemist, says, "There's your magnesium oil!" It'll be more watery than store-bought magnesium oil, but it works well and is less expensive.

Some women prefer to supplement with magnesium orally. Always speak to your healthcare provider before you begin to supplement. Some women cannot take magnesium orally at all; others need 2,000 milligrams a day. I take 1,200 milligrams to feel optimal. If you are taking thyroid medication, magnesium can block absorption. Wait at least four hours after taking your thyroid medication before consuming magnesium. (I wait seven hours.)

When we consume magnesium, it isn't always easily absorbed. Although magnesium oxide is inexpensive and widely available, I do not recommend this type because it is *very* poorly absorbed. It goes in your mouth and out in your stool. Magnesium citrate is more bio-available (more easily absorbed by the body), and it might be a good solution if you're also experiencing constipation. If not, magnesium citrate can cause loose stool, so use magnesium bis-glycinate instead.

Recommended: For rapid relief, I recommend running a hot bath, adding 2 cups of Epsom salts, and soaking for at least twenty minutes. Some women prefer a foot soak. Fill a bucket with hot water, add 1 cup of Epsom salts, and soak your feet for twenty to thirty minutes. Do this daily until you experience relief from cramps, and then three to four times a week afterward for maintenance.

Acid reflux

One of the benefits of fasting is that it can eliminate acid reflux, also commonly called heartburn, in the long run. But if you've struggled with acid reflux before, it can reoccur before it gets better when you start to fast. In normal digestion, a muscle at one end of the esophagus opens to let food into the stomach and then closes to prevent food and stomach juices from flowing back out. But with acid reflux, that muscle weakens and the acidic juices cause a burning sensation in the chest.

Researchers are unsure why people who experience reflux sometimes get it worse when they fast; it's possibly due to obesity, poor gut bacteria, and/or health issues such as kidney or liver dysfunction. Please check in with your doctor, and continue to take your medication for reflux when you are fasting. Most side effects subside within four to six weeks with consistent fasting and by using the tools recommended below.

Recommended: Stir freshly squeezed lemon juice into an 8-ounce glass of water several times a day, up to 3 tablespoons in total each day. Or do the same with up to 6 tablespoons of raw apple cider vinegar (or you can drink the apple cider vinegar straight). If you don't like the taste, add a pinch of salt. You can also have the lemon and the apple cider vinegar together if you prefer the flavor. Avoid bone broth and pickle juice, if you can.

Frequently Asked Questions: Tips and Tricks for Fasting Success

Questions about how to deal with side effects are the primary concerns many women have while fasting, but I also get asked lots of other questions, including which foods are best to eat when breaking a fast, whether it's safe to fast while taking medications, how to fast during stressful periods, and so on. Here I share the answers to these questions, along with other troubleshooting tips I've learned along the way with thousands of clients.

I'm taking thyroid medication. Can I fast?

Many women don't realize that the thyroid gland controls the efficiency of the gastrointestinal tract, and so an over- or underactive thyroid can create difficulties while fasting: diarrhea or loose stools can be a sign of hyperthyroidism (and Graves' disease), and chronic constipation is a sign of hypothyroidism (and Hashimoto's disease).

If you have Hashimoto's, the autoimmune disorder that can cause both underactive and overactive thyroid, check with your doctor before you begin any fast. Women with Hashimoto's often have the most issues with fasting, especially if they have a selenium deficiency. Because selenium plays a key role in metabolism, I encourage these women to talk to their doctor about taking 200 milligrams of selenium. It can be taken on an empty stomach at any time of day and needs to be taken regularly to build up in the system and help support the gastrointestinal tract, which reduces side effects of fasting.

One sign that any woman is becoming hyperthyroid and may need to lower her thyroid medication is loose stool that is not resolving within two to four weeks. If this is happening to you, then I recommend you consult a doctor or endocrinologist to get bloodwork done and see if you need to adjust your thyroid medication. I do not recommend adjusting thyroid medication without being seen by a medical professional.

I am taking nutritional supplements and medications that need to be consumed with food. Should I continue to take them when I fast? And how do I do this if I'm not eating?

Always work with your doctor, and never stop taking medication without their advice. Your doctor may want you to take certain medications and supplements every day, whether you are fasting or not, and some of those have to be taken with food. If that's the case, I have two strategies for you:

1 Stir 1 tablespoon of chia seeds or psyllium husks into an 8- or 16-ounce glass of water and let the mixture rest for about thirty minutes. You can drink this gel-like beverage to take your supplements and medications and still keep the integrity of your fast. This drink doesn't cause an insulin surge, so your body continues to experience the benefits of fasting and you can continue taking your medications or supplements.

2 Eat a cup of leafy greens, like romaine lettuce, and then take your supplements or medications. While consuming these greens means that you're not doing a "perfectly clean" fast, you're barely raising your insulin levels and so you'll be out of the fasting state for only a very short time. It's a far better approach than skipping your medications.

Note that vitamin C is fine to take on a fasting day and won't cause digestive tract issues for most women. Fat-soluble vitamins are hard to absorb when you're not eating, though, and some supplements, such as zinc, are very hard on your stomach if you don't take them with food. Please be attentive to what your body needs and what your doctor advises. It's more important to be consistent in your fasting than it is to become sick and in pain by taking supplements on an empty stomach. Work out a strategy with your doctor.

Will fasting cause me to become malnourished?

Not likely. Most North American women are *over*nourished—we have a tremendous amount of excess fuel in our bodies—but many of us *are* lacking in vital nutrients. The problem is not fasting; the problem is that a lot of the food that makes us overweight also has very low nutritional value. If you are consistent with your fasting protocol yet not losing any weight or making any progress toward resolving your metabolic issues, I recommend you get a SpectraCell micronutrient test. I have no affiliation with the company; I just like how easy their tests are to understand. The test will help you see which nutrients you are missing, and then you can either supplement or eat whole foods to balance them. Let's say, for example, that you're deficient in selenium, then you could eat a couple of Brazil nuts with each meal, or you could take one 200 milligram tablet of selenium per day with the Brazil nuts, to get yourself back to an optimal level.

Roshni's Story

When I first met Roshni, who was vegan, she was overweight, her skin was gray, and she was committed to consuming plant-based foods only. Her regular diet consisted of vegan pizza and vegan ice cream, but she had recently done a five-day fast and *gained* weight. She was heartbroken.

I asked her to do bloodwork with me, and we found that she was deeply deficient in essential nutrients—vitamins B_6 and B_{12}, magnesium, selenium, and iodine. To allow Roshni to gain control of her weight and normalize her blood sugars, the right protocol was to eat three meals a day for two months to replenish her nutrients, and then to try an intermittent fasting protocol of short fasts. We worked on her eating and used targeted supplementation.

After two months, I asked Roshni to do another round of bloodwork. She was finally well nourished, able to thrive, and ready to try fasting again. She had started to lose weight before she started fasting again because she'd learned how to eat as a vegan without losing all her nutrients. Roshni began doing two 48-hour fasts per week, a schedule that worked well with her two children, her husband, and her job. With her real-food diet and her fasting plan, she was no longer eating carbage. As a result, she managed to lose 60 pounds, reduce her supplementation, and feel great.

My life is *always* stressful. Any tips on how to fast while juggling a full-time job, family life, and community commitments?

Stress can involve positive emotions (like a wedding or a new baby) or negative emotions (like work stress or taking care of elderly parents), and it can also take a physical form (like an injury, infection, or poor sleep). If you are already under a lot of stress, consider whether you could fast at a different time. If you cannot clear time for a longer fast, focus on doing the best job you can with fat fasting (page 147) or time-restricted eating (page 154). Although you might not induce autophagy, you can satiate your body and reduce the number of hours you're stimulating insulin surges. Those are two benefits of fasting right there.

• TOP FIVE STRATEGIES FOR FASTING THROUGH A STRESSFUL TIME •

1 **Don't snack.** It's perfectly okay to eat almonds or dark chocolate, but make sure to eat them with your meals and not in between! Every time you snack—whether you're eating carbohydrates, fat, or protein—you cause your body to produce insulin. If you're struggling to lose weight or reverse your type 2 diabetes, then you already have too much insulin in your system, preventing fat loss and causing insulin resistance. If you don't snack, you won't add to the problem and cause more stress.

2 **Set aside a specific time for meal prep.** This tip is critical if you have to cook for others, especially children. You'll have healthy meals prepared ahead of time, so you're not tempted to serve up quick and easy processed foods. It also means spending less time in the kitchen, where you might be tempted to eat. I set aside a few hours on Sundays and Thursdays to prep my meals for the next few days while I listen to an inspirational podcast or audiobook. Eating healthy can be stress-free too!

3 **Stick to healthy natural fats.** If you are so stressed out that your appetite feels out of control, then try fat fasting. Only eating natural fats, such as avocados, bacon, and eggs, until you reach satiation leads your body to naturally start to fast. You'll feel full and not be tempted to snack or reach for treats, and you won't regret them later.

4 **Practice mindful eating.** Just as mindfulness meditation is important to help us manage stress, mindful eating (page 214)

is a priority for our overall health. Think about the long-term consequences of what you eat before you put it in your mouth. Potato chips might comfort you for a few minutes, but you'll feel terrible an hour later. Macadamia nuts leave you feeling satiated and without a nasty carb hangover.

5 **Join a group fasting and eating challenge in our community.** Our online Fasting Method community hosts weekly fasting and eating challenges led by me! We're very sensitive to what's going on in the world and we work with our members to find out what struggles they're having. Each weekly challenge is created with those struggles in mind. The idea is that you don't have to fast alone—you can do it with your friends in the community and draw on their support!

I need quick results. Will a five-day fast do it?

No. Maintaining consistency and seeing your fasting journey as a long-term change in how you eat will bring you long-lasting results. Fasting is *not* a case of "If one day is good for you, five days of it must be better." People who try this approach fail, console themselves with food, and end up heavier and with their highest blood sugar levels ever. When we crash and burn after trying to fast too much too soon, we return to our favorite foods and set ourselves up for poor health outcomes. If you want to do a longer fast, I recommend that you work up to it with shorter fasts first and that you work with an expert. You will meet your healing goals faster this way.

Please remember that multiple five-day fasts are not a base protocol for *anyone*. These longer fasts can make you crash and burn—and then never fast again. Use extended fasts one to four times a year at most for "deep cleaning," and stick to a regular schedule of two or three fasts each week the rest of the time.

I'm new to fasting.
What should I eat when I break my fast?

My main advice is to go slowly. Start by stirring 1 tablespoon of chia seeds or psyllium husks into an 8- or 16-ounce glass of water and let the mixture rest for about thirty minutes. Consume it half an hour before breaking your fast so it can absorb excess water in your gut and help your digestive tract as you reintroduce food.

Next, gently wake up your digestive tract with a tomato and cucumber salad with some olive oil and parsley. Parsley bulks up your stool, and tomato and cucumber are easy to digest. (I always tell my clients that eating an egg for breakfast is like someone punching you awake; it hits the digestive system hard.)

Follow your salad with cooked vegetables and poultry, including the skin of the chicken, which isn't too fatty despite what you may have been told. Remember, natural fats are good! Fish cooked in fat is another great option, as are leafy greens cooked in oils (not raw) for vegetarians and vegans. Half an avocado has a good amount of fiber that can bulk up the stool, and it's very satiating and unlikely to cause issues in the gut. If you consistently have trouble with your digestion, I suggest 2 tablespoons of chia or psyllium husks in water to start. Or use a full-fat yogurt or coconut kefir instead of water.

I hear protein can cause side effects when fasting.
Is that true?

Some experts say that protein is everything. Others suggest that we eat too much of it. When we look at the science, the jury is out—there is data supporting both theories.

In my clinical practice, when women with insulin resistance and type 2 diabetes eat too much protein, they notice their blood sugar goes up. I recommend that instead of having a 12-ounce steak, they elect to have an 8-ounce steak. Once these clients fast for a little bit and their metabolic levels go *up*, they become more active and want to go hiking or play golf or go to the gym. Their body composition dramatically shifts, and they have more lean mass, and so then they do need more protein. That's when I suggest they try the 12-ounce steak.

In contrast, if a woman is not getting enough protein on eating days, it's *very* hard to fast. I see women get into fasting plateaus: they're not able to fast anymore because they're experiencing side effects. Symptoms of low protein are brain fog, increased sugar cravings, and hair loss. Increasing protein intake (usually by a couple of ounces of meat, for example) on an eating day is the solution.

The bottom line is that at the start of your journey, you may not tolerate protein, but that may change.

I've tried a few fasts, and I always get cravings midafternoon. Is there a way to stop them?

I've heard tens of thousands of times that the 4 p.m. witching hour is the problem time of day for many women. This is because the intense stress of juggling many demands early in the day causes our adrenal glands to continuously produce cortisol. The higher our cortisol levels go, the more fatigued our adrenal glands become and the more we crave sugar. For most women, this peak occurs around 4 p.m. Sugar stimulates the release of cortisol, which gives us the energy to deal with our stress.

If you take salt every two to four hours starting in the morning, you give your adrenal glands a big hug while trying to get the kids to school, dealing with your email inbox, or juggling meetings and urgent work requests—or all of those at once! Sodium is the number one life support for your adrenal glands, decreasing the amount of cortisol released in response to stress. How much salt you take depends on your level of insulin resistance.

If you have high insulin resistance, your body holds onto sodium and you might not need to take much salt. But six weeks down the road of your fasting journey, your insulin levels may have come down so much that you're not holding sodium in your body and fasting becomes impossible. When you find yourself experiencing fatigue, headaches, and 4 p.m. cravings, have a little sodium every four hours. Increase that to every two hours as you proceed along your fasting journey.

I've been losing weight by fasting, but it's not working any more. What am I doing wrong?

You've hit a plateau, and it's completely normal. Whether you're no longer losing weight, suddenly ravenously hungry during the fast, or having increased side effects, everyone stalls at some point on their fasting journey. To get past this stage, try one or more of these strategies.

1 **Change the fasting protocol you've been using.** If you've been using a 16/8 or a 18/6 fast, try a longer fast or three fasts a week. If you've been doing three 42-hour fasts a week, try two 48-hour fasts a week to give you more time in a deeper fat burning state. If you've plateaued using a longer fast, try eating more or doing three 24-hour fasts a week instead.

2 **Show up for your fasts as if they're therapeutic treatments.** They are. The more consistent you are, the better the results will be.

3 **Make sure you're supplementing with salt and magnesium.** Keeping your electrolytes in balance will keep your metabolism in peak working order. (See page 184.)

4 **Don't snack *ever*.** Eating triggers insulin and moves you from fat burning to fat storing. Remember that when you are fasting, you are healing.

5 **Try some new eating strategies.** How you eat (see Chapter 12) can change your relationship with food and help you better recognize when you are satiated.

Will intermittent fasting interfere with my menstrual cycle or make me infertile?

No. Fasting is more likely to regulate your cycle and reduce the symptoms of PMS dramatically! Like many of the women I've worked with, I was scared to fast at first, wondering how it would affect my fertility. But then I realized that only recently have we been able to go to the refrigerator and pull out a dozen eggs or go to the cupboard and grab a box of cereal. For centuries, we had to hunt and gather and that meant periods of scarcity, which is like enforced intermittent fasting. Women obviously had no issues reproducing or else I wouldn't be here and neither would you.

For the first two months of fasting, most women report delayed menstrual cycles. And many still have the cramping, bloating, cravings, and irritability that they've always had. The good news is that these symptoms don't get worse before they get better, despite all the hormonal changes that are occurring. Don't fast when your body or life isn't cooperating. Do your best to fat fast or stick to a low carb, high healthy fat approach for the first few months.

Around months three and four, most of the physical and emotional side effects of PMS start to diminish greatly. Menstrual timing starts to regulate whether you've had extremely or mildly irregular periods in the past. Even women who haven't had periods in nearly two years start to experience normal cycles within the first six months of fasting—it's incredible! Women report that their appetite is still strong, but the cravings for unhealthy processed carbs have diminished significantly. I still encourage fat fasting during this time.

The magic seems to happen by month six. The side effects of PMS are a distant memory, and you feel in control of your diet. This is when I suggest women start to actively fast during their period. They start to notice weight loss during their periods rather than weight gain! And to add to all of the goodness, women often report that days one through seven of their cycle are the easiest days for them to fast every month.

Can fasting help me lose the weight I'm gaining through menopause and help with other menopausal changes?

Yes. Many women going through menopause believe they're doomed when it comes to losing weight. I've had the privilege of working with thousands of women going through "the change," and I'll be the first to say losing weight during this period isn't easy. But it isn't impossible either. In fact, women can get amazing results during menopause by following some basic fasting principles. Consistency, cutting out snacking, and patience are your best friends. I have yet to work with a single woman who hasn't been able to lose weight, but it has taken a lot of trial and error to figure out protocols that really work, and you must be diligent about following them.

Some women report that fasting helps boost sexual desire and increase vaginal wetness. Every now and then, a woman reports that her gray hair has disappeared or that she has fewer or less intense hot flashes. These symptoms rarely go away completely, but they do improve. Studies have also shown that fasting can help improve bone health, including osteoporosis.[2]

How do I manage exercise while fasting?

Many clients worry about how to balance exercise with fasting so they don't feel exhausted or drained. When they feel hungry after a workout, they think that they need glucose or protein. In fact, we need to replenish our *sodium levels*. During a workout, we lose about half a teaspoon of salt through sweat every half an hour. One way to replenish sodium is to hydrate well before you work out. I recommend mixing half a teaspoon of salt into a liter of water. By drinking the slightly salted water ninety minutes before training, you give your body time to absorb it, optimize for exercise, and have time to use the bathroom. You're ready to work out even if it's a fasting day—and it feels easy and fun!

FASTING IS A simple way to change your relationship with food and to heal your body. The questions that I've answered for you in this chapter are the ones I hear most often, but other questions do arise. If you encounter any side effects or need help troubleshooting, and your question isn't answered here, please visit my online platform to find more specific answers. I also invite you to join my Facebook group, where women connect to discuss their own unique fasting journeys.

In the next chapter, we look at strategies to incorporate fasting into your life as you progress on your journey. By now, you've been fasting for a while, and you've found solutions to hurdles that have arisen—and you know to seek me out online to help you with any stumbles. The next part of the book shares everything I've learned to help make day-to-day fasting something that you manage easily and successfully.

Chapter 11 Takeaways

- Many side effects of fasting are caused by our electrolytes being out of balance. Supplementing with sodium and some magnesium prevents us from shedding other essential electrolytes, and that keeps our body working efficiently.

- Learning from other women, online and in person, and supporting each other's fasting journeys helps all of us get through any side effects or trouble spots we may encounter.

Tips and Tricks for Building a Healthy Relationship With Food

• • • • •

"Fasting today makes the food good tomorrow."
GERMAN PROVERB

WE'VE TALKED THROUGHOUT the book about thinking of fasting as healing. In this chapter, I want you to start thinking more deeply about eating days being *rebuilding* days. The types of foods we consume, and how we consume those foods, affects our healing journey. Avocados, for example, cause different hormonal responses than sugary cereal, as we know. Keep that avocado in mind, and the hormonal response it causes as we explore the different roles food plays in our lives. We often think of food as our best friend: comforting us, being there for us. But now I want you to think of food as fuel: for your journey to health.

In this chapter, there are two main topics. The first is the physical art of how to eat—which is all about understanding when you're full and not full. This means learning how to interpret your bodily sensations, your hormones, and the messages being sent. The second part is about what to eat. A lot of people come to fasting and think that *what* to eat is most important, but from my perspective, the most important part is *how* to eat.

How to Eat: Three Ways to Curb Grazing and Overeating to Keep Insulin Low

When I work with clients on eating and food choices, they expect lots of recipes. They're thinking in terms of *what* to eat. I prefer to begin with *how* to eat. I usually start by asking them what they feel when they finish a meal. Take a moment to ask yourself these questions and jot down your answers:

- Do you ever feel full?

- What does feeling full *feel* like?

If you're like a lot of my clients, you answered *No* or *I don't know*. Many people never feel full or know the feeling of satiation. And that is a big reason for overeating.

Leptin is our primary satiation hormone. When we're full, our fat cells release leptin, which travels through the bloodstream to our brain where our leptin receptors are. The brain then sends the message to stop eating and start burning fat. But many people have no idea what it feels like to feel full because *leptin never reaches their leptin receptors*. Why not? Because insulin and inflammation get in the way. When the body contains lots of leptin but the brain doesn't receive the signal, there is leptin resistance.

Chronic stress can lead to inflammation. For many people, a diet high in grains and dairy causes a lot of inflammation. And all that inflammation prevents leptin from binding with its receptors. This prevents proper hormonal signaling to indicate when we've consumed enough. The result? It's impossible to ever feel full.

So, we eat more.

And more.

And the cycle of inflammation continues.

There's also another reason that many women don't know what satiation feels like, and it's psychological. Many of us started dieting in middle school, and many of us have followed at least one calorie-restriction diet—and often dozens or even hundreds. We've eaten the special branded diet foods, we've counted the points or calories, but we've never focused on whether or not we felt full. Most calorie-restriction diets do not recommend eating satiating foods; they focus on low-calorie foods, which drive insulin production too. For many women, the idea of satiation has been tangled up with the deprivation model of dieting—feeling full is considered a bad thing.

We have a whole population of women who are terrified to gain weight, and they associate feeling full with gaining weight. Ninety-five percent of the women who come into my program have no idea if they are full or not, if they need to eat more or not.

Learn to recognize satiation: The ninety-minute eating strategy

I want you to picture eating an avocado: feeling its cool creamy flesh in your mouth, savoring its earthy, slightly nutty or buttery flavor. How do you feel? Notice what it tastes like in your mind. Avocados suppress insulin and don't cause inflammation, which means that leptin gets to its receptors and you feel full. Think about your hormonal response and this feeling of satiation as you read on.

When clients come to me not knowing how to determine if they feel full, I introduce the ninety-minute eating strategy. For many people, this simple approach to eating transforms their relationship with food after years of dieting and misery. I ask people to think of each meal as having three thirty-minute chunks.

THE NINETY-MINUTE EATING STRATEGY

First 30 minutes	Eat your meal.
Second 30 minutes	Sit and digest.
Third 30 minutes	Assess and evaluate if you are still hungry.

In the first thirty minutes, eat your meal. In the second thirty minutes, give your body the time it needs to digest and your hormones need to send the message of fullness. Do not eat or drink anything more during these thirty minutes. This pause helps ensure you don't get *too* full because of overeating. You can sit at the table and socialize during this time or resume light work, although try not to do anything overly physical because you want to pay attention to your body.

In the third thirty minutes, think about that feeling of satiation from eating an avocado. Is that how you feel? If yes, you've eaten a meal that is well designed for you, and you've had enough fat and carbs. Great. If you are still hungry, ask yourself, "What am I craving?" Fat, sweetness, carbs? Once you've determined what you are craving, *eat more of that*. My clients are so surprised when I say this, but it's crucial that you top up your food and help yourself truly feel full in this third thirty-minute period.

This strategy helps many women learn when they are satiated, and it's a tool I recommend you come back to over and over again throughout your fasting journey as your relationship with food changes.

Remember when I talked about the nineteen different metabolic versions of myself? I started out as a very sick individual who would look at a pile of laundry and cry. Doctors told me I couldn't have children because of my PCOS. I had type 2 diabetes and fatty liver disease. Then I became Megan who desired more physical activity, became more active, and was on a path to wellness. That Megan had a different set of nutritional needs. Each time I had a new metabolic persona, I hit a wall where my hunger was through the roof when I was fasting. Suddenly I'd have sugar cravings. Once I had a craving for a date cookie—even when I had type 2 diabetes, I never wanted to eat those; I don't like them! But that metabolic version of me wanted that cookie.

Cravings and plateaus are a sign that you need to reassess if you need more fat fuel to support your increased physical activity or more protein to support your body. A deficiency in protein makes you crave sweet things, for example. The key is not to focus on the specific type of protein but on how much.

Throughout your healing journey, you'll experience these changes, and that's when the ninety-minute eating strategy is useful. Return to eating mindfully, and design your own ideal meal. What you're doing in this process is learning how much and what types of food your body needs in the first meal—that first thirty minutes—so that eventually you don't have to eat in that third period of thirty minutes. Reevaluate and reevaluate. I encourage you to keep coming back to this strategy. It is a proven way to help you get to know your body, and your new body, as you progress on your metabolic journey.

• EXPERT TIP •

Be sure to use the ninety-minute eating strategy properly. Stop eating after the first thirty minutes, whether or not you have finished all the food on your plate. Then wait a full thirty minutes before you assess if you're still hungry. It takes at least twenty minutes for leptin to get to the receptors in your brain, and so it's crucial to take this time, be mindful, and teach yourself how to be satiated, wherever you are on your fasting journey.

Finally, do not automatically use the third thirty minutes to consume. The idea is to learn what to eat in that first period and eventually shrink the mealtime to between thirty-five and forty minutes total. The pause after you've eaten is for you to receive that hormonal response to the food you've eaten, not to eat some more!

Exceptions to the ninety-minute eating strategy

- Give yourself grace when you're experiencing a lot of stress. Sometimes, on stressful days, you'll be hungrier, and the ninety-minute eating strategy may not be useful for you then. Try the ninety-minute eating strategy the next day, or a few days later when you have a better window.

- Another time to give yourself grace is during a holiday period when you've gathered with family and friends. It's important to enjoy eating with our communities. Set the timer on your watch for ninety minutes, and savor the food and the company. After the ninety minutes, stop eating. This way you avoid conflict and social discomfort, and you support your health journey and your learning about satiety. In my family, for example, we have food out all day long on Christmas: we start eating in the morning, keep going all day long, and then have a huge dinner. I might

213

enjoy the meat and cheese hors d'oeuvres over ninety minutes in the morning and then stop eating and wait for the holiday meal. Then I do the same thing at dinner: eat turkey and vegetables over ninety minutes and then stop.

Learn to eat in timed windows: Mini-fasting

If you're like me and love to snack, mini-fasting can help curb the urge to graze throughout your eating days. Grazing for hours causes insulin secretion, which leads to insulin resistance, which leads to obesity and type 2 diabetes. Every time we eat, even low-carb foods, we produce insulin. A little bit here and a little bit there adds up to a *lot* of insulin. And our whole goal is to reduce the amount of insulin we're secreting overall, every day. Cutting out snacking was the most critical step in optimizing my weight loss and maintaining my health. Remember, I was diagnosed with type 2 diabetes; to stay well, I need to make sure my body isn't constantly producing insulin.

To ensure you aren't snacking or grazing on your rebuilding days, eat two to three meals and fast between those eating windows. You eat lunch, say, from 1 to 2 p.m., then dinner from 6 to 7 p.m. And if you can, keep your meals to around thirty-five minutes. Between lunch and dinner, from 2 to 6 p.m., you mini-fast. In an ideal world, you'd have a 4-hour mini-fast, and not more than 6 hours, between your meals.

I like to do group challenges with clients where the goal isn't the number of fasting days but the number of hours you're not eating food between meals. This approach gamifies eating days and helps participants have fun, while their body rebuilds. If snacking is a problem for you, try something similar so you aren't causing insulin secretion multiple times throughout the day.

Learn to engage your parasympathetic response: Mindful eating

Many of us eat while doing something else, which means that we're not paying attention to our food at all. Mindless eating leads to poor food choices, overeating, and poor digestion. Simply paying a bit more attention when we're eating can make a big difference to our health.

We don't think a lot about our digestion, unless it's working poorly and causing us pain. Our digestion is run by the autonomic nervous system, a two-part system that controls involuntary actions in the body. The first part is our sympathetic nervous system (SNS); the second is our parasympathetic nervous system (PNS).

We know our SNS well because when we feel stress—facing a lion or bear, say, in prehistoric times, or dealing with a slew of urgent emails in modern times—our fight-or-flight response is activated. Our body goes into survival mode, preparing to fight and shutting off digestion. The body turns on our fat-storing mode since it isn't sure when we're going to be fed again. When our attention is elsewhere—whether on a new baby, a cute dog video, a tragic news story, or a recent loss—and not on our food, we trigger our sympathetic nervous system. Our body interprets that distraction as a *stress response*, and we don't absorb nutrients, which leads to digestive issues.

Most of us know much less about the parasympathetic nervous system, otherwise known as our rest-and-digest system. After danger has passed or when there is no stress or distraction, our heart rate slows, our blood pressure drops, and our body turns on our metabolism so we can absorb nutrients and begin healing and repairing our cells again. There's only one scenario in which we can be distracted and have a parasympathetic response, and that is when we're engaging with a group of people (say, around a dinner table conversing and enjoying a meal with friends). We have a parasympathetic response, which is relaxing and means that our food is digesting properly.

The key to engaging the parasympathetic nervous system is to be relaxed and focused on what we are eating. If you live and eat alone, I encourage you to play nice music in the background, or eat outside for the pleasant sounds of wind and birds, which is relaxing for our system. I encourage you to sit down and focus on your meal, eat in a place specifically designated for eating (not at your desk), and put away your phone, your work, and any other distractions.

People struggle to learn how to eat mindfully. But it's the same as learning how to be mindful when meditating. You learn to focus on your breath when you are meditating, and I suggest that you count your chews to help focus on your food. Optimally, you should chew eighteen times before you swallow. That can be a lot for people to start with, so try ten chews, then build up to eighteen. When you have practiced this approach, it gets easier to eat mindfully and prompt a parasympathetic response.

• EXPERT TIP •

Mindful eating is the most difficult practice for clients to adopt, but when I challenge groups to try mindful eating for two weeks, they are astonished by the results. They lose more weight, have better bowel movements, and no longer feel bloated. There is a huge shift that can make or break our fasting results.

To start, focus on the textures, combinations, and tastes of your food. How does broccoli taste with salmon, for example, and how is that different when you eat broccoli on its own? Try one of these prompts to guide your mindful eating journey.

1 Focus on the food you most enjoy in this meal.

2 Listen to the sound of your cutlery as you cut your food. What other sounds can you hear?

3 How is this meal making you feel?

I wanted us to think about *how* to eat before we look at *what* to eat, because how we eat is crucial to our relationship with food. It's much easier to select healthful foods when you're thinking about rebuilding and when you really understand when you're satiated or still hungry. Now, we'll explore what foods are best for you as you fuel your body for your life.

What to Eat: How to Choose the Right Diet for *You*

In Chapter 4, we looked at the main components of food—carbohydrates, proteins, and natural fats—and their effects on the body. And we know that by reducing the number of refined carbohydrates and increasing natural fats, we lower insulin secretion. In general, people are coming around to the fact that sugar is truly the dietary demon and that a lot of our weight gain and health issues have to do with the processed and refined sugars we consume. Historically, we blamed fat for what sugar did, but we're starting to understand that error and move toward diets based on more ancestral ways of eating.

Let's look at some of the most popular current diets, whether these help or hinder our ability to reduce insulin, and how to determine what foods might be best for you.

Paleo diet

On this popular diet, people eat meat, fish, seafood, any vegetables—especially leafy greens—and some fruits, along with nuts and seeds. Some people include pasteurized dairy products, and others include no dairy at all. Paleo is a liberal approach to whole-food-based eating from an ancestral perspective. In a liberal low-carb diet, like Paleo, you would consume no more than 100 grams of carbs per day. (In a moderate one, it would be 50 grams of carbs per day.)

Both the American Diabetes Association and the American Heart Association recognize low-carb diets, such as Paleo, as safe ways to manage heart disease and diabetes. These diets are gaining in popularity as people see health changes when they reduce grains and cut out sugars.

Keto diet

With a keto diet, which has also become a very popular way to eat, people eat mostly healthy natural fats and a moderate amount of protein. Their carbohydrate intake is very low because virtually every high-carb food is reduced or eliminated from the diet. About 70 percent of calories in this diet come from natural fats, 20 percent from protein, and 10 percent from carbs. A keto diet has no more than about 20 grams of carbs per day.

The Charlie Foundation has funded a lot of medical research on the benefits of ketogenic therapies. People who follow a keto diet are in a constant state of ketosis; fat becomes the primary fuel source for the body, instead of glucose. This is the goal. When the body does not have glucose to burn for fuel, it uses ketones and fatty acids.

Plant-based diet

In a plant-based diet, people eat vegetables, nuts, seeds, legumes, and lentils. Many people believe that plant-based eating and a Paleo diet are incompatible, but that's not the case. The key is to find which foods work for you. Some people eat moderate amounts of gluten-free grains, such as millet, buckwheat, amaranth, quinoa, teff, and rice (black, wild, or red). You can try eating small servings of legumes—such as black soybeans, peas, green beans, and lentils—and if you don't experience any symptoms of gastric distress (bloating or abdominal pain), you can continue to consume them. Most importantly, to stay within a low-carb approach, watch your portion size of starchy vegetables, gluten-free grains, and legumes and lentils. Limit your intake of these foods to one-quarter of your dish. Use non-starchy fibrous vegetables, like leafy greens and vegetables that grow above the ground, to make up the balance. Finally, don't shy away from fat! Excellent sources of plant-based fats are olives, avocados, coconuts, and their fats.

Choose any variation of a low-carb diet

Any low-carb approach is usually a good choice for your rebuilding days, especially for anyone dealing with metabolic issues, autoimmune issues, inflammation, or obesity. At the start of your health journey, you may need to keep your carbs very low (keto diet) so that you feel optimal. As your body heals from insulin resistance and you become more active, you can eat more carbs and still stay in a primarily fat-fueling state. This ability to adapt is known as metabolic flexibility. When I started fasting, I ate 20 grams of carbs total on my rebuilding days, but now I can consume 100 grams of carbs a day and I'm still primarily in a fat-fueling state. Apps like Carb Manager, Cronometer, and MyFitnessPal can help you track the number of carbs you consume in a day.

Consider increasing your carbs later in your healing journey

Many women are afraid to go back to eating carbs because this macronutrient has become so demonized. But they often reach a plateau trying to lose the last 15 to 20 pounds, and that's when they can benefit greatly from introducing *more* carbs into their diet. Some clients who are stuck in this anti-carb thinking go on vacation, eat more carbs, and are surprised to find they *lose* weight. Because their bodies are no longer insulin resistant, eating carbs supports adrenal function and optimizes their hormonal function. This step always occurs later in the healing journey—and is very individual. I generally recommend that women at this stage of their fasting journey consume around 100 grams of carbs twice a week.

Eat your carbs "dressed"

Not all carbs are created equal. Some create a lot of inflammation in the body—like pizza, cake, and cookies! These are often called "bad" carbs, or carbage, and we want to avoid them. But even "good" carbs—natural whole foods such as sweet potatoes, berries, quinoa, and legumes—can cause an insulin spike. The term I use to help clients think about this phenomenon in a healthful way comes from dietician and nutritionist Lily Nichols who describes the importance of having your carbs *naked* or *dressed*.[1]

If you eat a potato on its own—naked—the potato will be rapidly digested, causing an insulin spike. If you eat it with other food, maybe with vinegar or other food on your plate, you dress it. When you dress up a carbohydrate, you change its chemical composition. The potatoes goes into your belly along with fat, fiber, and protein. The vinegar slows digestion. In other words, mixing the potato with other foods stops the glucose spike, slows digestion, and helps your body absorb the carbs healthfully.

You can choose to have your healthy carbs in a healthy fashion by *dressing* them. If you have a handful of berries by themselves, for example, you spike your glucose. But if you eat those berries with coconut cream, chia seeds, and crushed nuts, you help the body digest the carbs well.

Save your carbs for last

I like this analogy: if you're potting a plant, you might put rocks at the bottom, then soil, then the plant. In the same way, think about layering foods when you eat. The smallest insulin response comes from fats, so eat them *first* to help your satiation response and reduce your hunger. Then eat the protein. And finish up with the carbs.

My Story

I'd made so much progress and restricted carbs for so long that when the first Thanksgiving in my fasting journey rolled around, I promised myself I was going to eat my mother's roasted potatoes. I hadn't eaten potatoes for months at this point! I was like a kid with dessert before supper. In a semifasted state, I ate potatoes first, stuffing them into my empty belly. The potatoes rapidly digested, I had a massive insulin spike, and my body started to produce ghrelin—the hunger hormone—in response.

I ate more potatoes, and then bread, and I was so hungry I wanted to eat everything. I ate and ate and had a very delayed satiation response. I felt terrible, gained a lot of water weight, and it took days to get my hormones re-regulated. I had to fat fast to calm my inflammation!

At Christmas that same year, I was determined to not make the same mistake. I ate my turkey, sprouts, and salad with some vinegar. I made sure to eat the potatoes last. I parented myself: I ate fats followed by proteins, and I had a strong hormonal satiation response. I only ate half the potatoes. For the first time in my life, I left potatoes on my plate! I enjoyed my meal and my day so much. Saving the carbs for the end really helps manage the body's hormonal response.

What to Eat: How to Adapt in Social Situations, on Vacation, and After Weight-Loss Surgery

Adapting your eating strategies at home or with close family for a special occasion can take some planning, but dealing with public situations, longer periods away from home, or postoperative recovery can sometimes seem challenging and overwhelming. Plan ahead to deal with these situations, and you'll feel more prepared when they arise. Think about what you might say ahead of time, or talk with your loved ones so they know what to expect, though sometimes people respond in unhelpful ways. Here's some advice to help you plan and navigate this new phase in your life.

Social situations: Take the focus off fasting

Going for coffee or a drink or grabbing a bite to eat is a big part of how we connect with friends or work colleagues. If you're confident letting others know that you're carefully choosing your foods or fasting, that's great. But many women find the social pressure in these situations difficult to manage. How often have you heard people say, "Have cake! It's my birthday!" or "Have a drink! We're celebrating!"? In these situations, you have a couple of options: move the conversation away from fasting to avoid the questions and possible judgment, or choose a non-food-focused activity so that the topic of food or fasting doesn't come up at all.

When I first met the man who became my husband, he lived in San Francisco. I visited him from Toronto every three weeks. People come to San Fran to eat because the food is incredible! So, I used my time in Toronto to fast and eat "clean," and when I was in San Francisco I'd enjoy meals with friends and go to wineries in Napa or Sonoma. Both my husband and I lost weight during that time. Then my husband moved to Toronto. Our whole dating life, all of our activities together, were centered on eating at restaurants and connecting with each other and friends over food. We had no clean eating time, and we gained 12 pounds *each*!

We sat down and came up ways to connect other than over food. We chose puzzles and board games. If I was fasting, we'd drink tea and play a board game after he had eaten. In the summer, we'd go for hikes and explore outdoors. Our close friends love to eat and party, but we found that they also love to bike. Now we go for bike rides with one of our favorite couples, instead of out for drinks. We ride trails, have a healthy lunch stop, and enjoy spending time together in a way that suits all of us. My best friend and I used to go for supper together on Fridays, but we switched that to weekly pedicures, which both of us love so much more! Instead of baking with my female cousins around the holidays, we've created a healthier ritual: we play games together. And we invite the male cousins who love being a part of this new tradition.

Sometimes, though, it's not possible to avoid a social situation involving food. And when people find out that you're fasting, they can be very curious and intense about it. That can be uncomfortable, and some women feel compelled to break their fast just to avoid the questioning. Dr. Fung says the first rule of fasting is not to talk about it. But I recommend having a ready answer. You might say, "I'm doing the Whole30 diet!" Or my best friend suggests, "I'm on a dry month." Both of these responses are socially acceptable answers to questions that may challenge your fasting journey.

Suann's Story

Suann had a long-standing tradition of going to lunch with her close friends. Soon after she told her friends she had begun a fasting journey for weight loss and type 2 diabetes, they stopped inviting her to join them. They were uncomfortable with her choice to fast, even though Suann felt she could modify her fasting schedule to have lunch with them. She didn't want to have to choose between her health and her friends.

When Suann next came to see me, we came up with other ways she might connect with her friends. She decided to go for walks with them, which meant they talked about the cherry blossoms they saw or the new part of town they explored rather than about fasting or their eating differences. Their connection has become strong again, and her friends no longer make her feel guilty for electing to fast.

Suann has been consistently following the two 48-hour fasts a week protocol. She is now close to her goal of fully reversing her diabetes and losing the weight she intended to.

Vacations: Avoid snacks and stick to your eating strategies

If you're on holiday at an all-inclusive beach resort or on a cruise ship where there is constant access to food and sugary alcoholic drinks, you're at risk of gaining weight due to the abundance of food. But I don't recommend that you try to do a 16- or 24-hour fast on vacation either, because if you're out on the hot sunny beach, you're likely to get dehydrated and make poor food choices. I usually encourage clients in this situation to eat a breakfast rich in electrolytes and high in healthy fats and protein: some avocado, salmon, and bacon for example. Try mini-fasting, eating mindfully, or using the ninety-minute eating strategy. Clients sometimes lose weight on vacation when they follow this advice because they are better satiated and their electrolytes are better supported in the heat.

If you're on a sightseeing trip that's more active, it's usually hard to overeat because you're taking in everything there is to see in, say, Paris or on the Amalfi Coast. You may be eating two wonderful meals each day, but you often don't have a kitchen in your room or access to snacks, so you tend to lose weight during the vacation because your body is well sated and you're getting so much exercise. By not snacking or grazing, true time-restricted eating is a side benefit of all the sightseeing, and you're likely to improve your health—even if you're eating all those big, delicious meals. I've seen this result so many times; it truly reaffirms to me the importance of *never* snacking!

After weight-loss surgery: Eat smaller meals

Women who have had gastric bypass surgery (where the stomach is made smaller) or lap-band surgery (where a band is placed around the stomach to reduce its capacity and slow digestion) often find that they gain weight as time goes by. This can be extremely dispiriting, and women who come to me having regained the weight they lost during the surgery are often struggling with the emotions they have around managing their weight. Many of these women also have a lot of gastric distress when they eat, which can make fasting problematic.

In general, we need to eat larger meals when we break our fasts, eating mindfully until we're satiated. But with lap-band surgery, larger meals can be very uncomfortable. And with gastric bypass surgery, it can be very dangerous to eat a lot in one meal; it overstrains the stomach and can burst the stitches, leading to hospitalization. A lot of these women can't get enough nutrients through their food and are nutrient deficient.

In my clinical experience, the best fasting protocol for women who've had weight-loss surgery is three 36-hour fasts a week. You eat three smaller meals on eating (rebuilding) days, which is tolerable for the digestive system. Another strategy I recommend is three 42-hour fasts each week but with *three small meals* during a 6-hour window rather than the two larger meals typical in this protocol. I do not recommend the 48-hour fasting protocol because you eat only one meal, which can be uncomfortable or dangerous for the gastric system and makes it difficult to get enough nutrients. If you do try a longer fast with one meal to break it, I recommend eating soup; if that causes distress to the stomach, smoothies work well instead.

Cyndy's Story

The average person tries 126 diets in their lifetime.[2] Cyndy was one of those people. She had tried all the well-known diets, and she'd gained and lost the same 100 pounds over and over again. Finally, her doctor recommended lap-band surgery; the idea was that she would eat less and less often—like with intermittent fasting, but in her case with a huge surgery.

Cyndy had the surgery and initially lost the weight, but after she'd healed from the surgery, she went back to her old eating habits. She ate all the time and all the wrong things—and soon she gained back all of the weight plus *more*.

When Cyndy came to see me, I recommended three 36-hour fasts a week. She started fasting and she lost 160 pounds over eighteen months through fasting and real food nutrition. She was able to lose the lap band and has maintained a healthy weight ever since.

This is a very common story when it comes to women and weight-loss surgeries: they can't eat much in the short term after surgery, and when they can eat again, they gain all the weight back. However, if they begin fasting, learn to cut out snacks, and eat mindfully, they are able to get the lap band removed and maintain their weight loss.

We've looked at all sorts of ways to incorporate fasting into your life, strategies to relearn how to eat healthfully and mindfully, and specific guidance for certain individuals during their fasting journey. In the final chapter of the book, we turn to making fasting and healthy eating a lifelong habit.

Chapter 12 Takeaways

- The ninety-minute eating strategy is my secret weapon for everyone on their fasting journey. Review and practice it over and over to relearn satiation as your body changes.

- Mini-fasting is a very useful tool to maintain health, manage stressful situations, and ensure we enjoy vacations while we live with a new approach to food.

- When we eat while doing something else, we fail to activate our parasympathetic nervous system and do not digest our food well. Mindful eating will make a big difference to your fasting progress.

- Make sure to eat nutritious foods and to minimize your carbs, adjusting as you progress through your fasting journey. When traveling, consider eating healthy breakfasts so you don't get dehydrated.

- If you have had gastric surgery, use a fasting protocol that allows you to eat smaller meals rather than one large meal. Break your fast with soups or smoothies, which are easier to digest.

- The tools and strategies in this chapter are always here for you to refer to. They have worked for thousands of my clients and are designed to help women like you as you fast.

How to Make Fasting and Healthy Eating a Lifelong Habit

• • • • •

"Periodic fasting can help clear up the mind and strengthen the body and the spirit."
EZRA TAFT BENSON

MANY WOMEN HAVE spent a lifetime dedicated to weight loss without long-term success. If this is you, you may begin to panic as your body changes after months of fasting and you start to reach your goals—losing weight, healing, reversing type 2 diabetes. You may fear that you'll regain weight as you have with every diet in your life. You may think that weight loss is not sustainable. Because fasting is an entirely different experience, it can be confusing to navigate our new body (and our perceptions of it), to think about developing a new mindset to manage (rather than lose) weight, and to incorporate our new eating and fasting behaviors into our life for the long term. At this stage of the fasting journey, I get asked three things most often:

1   How do I know I'm at my goal?

2   What type of fasting will maintain my goal?

3   What type of food will maintain my goal?

I'll answer each of these questions to help you avoid the most common mistakes I see my clients make. This chapter will also give you confidence that you can maintain good health in the long term, even if you're not perfect 100 percent of the time. Fasting is a journey: there are times when you coast along smoothly, and there will be bumps in the road. It's how you respond to those bumps that makes the difference. Spend some time thinking about your healing mindset, and set yourself the goal of celebrating your body for all the wonderful things it does for you. If you gain a bit of weight or your blood sugar levels start to rise, don't panic. Set a healing intention, and trust that you can make good dietary and fasting choices to bring your body back to balance.

How Do I Know I'm at My Goal?

When we think about reaching a goal, we often measure success quantitatively. In other words, we look at the numbers—and for many of my clients, that means blood markers for type 2 diabetes and body mass for obesity. Those numbers can be helpful for understanding the changes taking place in the body, and we'll look at them in a moment. But building a healthy relationship with your body is not only about the numbers. It's about how we feel in our body. I call those the *human moments*.

For those with type 2 diabetes, the human moment is a normal glucose response. That is, after we eat, blood glucose naturally rises. If it comes down within a couple of hours, that's a normal response, and that's a helpful and valid healing goal. For those who are obese, the human moments are a healthy body weight set point and body composition. Our *body weight set point* is the mass at which our body reaches homeostasis. Remember our resting metabolic rate? Our RMR revs up or slows down to keep us at that set point, and fasting can lower the body weight at which that homeostasis occurs. We also want a body composition that sees fat evenly distributed across the body rather than deposited around the internal organs. Make the human moments your new healing goals.

Type 2 diabetes

No magical test can tell you if you've reversed your type 2 diabetes, though several blood markers can confirm that you're on the right path. Your doctor will want to see that:

1 Your hemoglobin A1C is in the optimal range of 4.5 to 5.2 percent

2 Your triglyceride levels are under 100mg/dL or 1 mmol/L

3 Your ratio of good cholesterol (high-density lipoproteins, or HDL) to triglyceride levels should be less than 1

These markers signal that you're going in the right direction, but even as these numbers improve, it doesn't mean that your insulin resistance has gone.

One marker that people with type 2 diabetes are taught to monitor is their HOMA-IR (homeostatic assessment of insulin resistance), which calculates how much insulin your body needs to make to control your blood sugar levels. In my clinical experience, this marker goes up and down very drastically. I used to check HOMA-IR every month in my patients, and I found that stress—a fight with a partner, a car accident, even a difficult workday—often elevated this marker, making it hard to assess with any certainty if type 2 diabetes was being reversed. I no longer recommend checking this marker or using it as a measure of success.

I do recommend that you look at A1C, triglycerides, and your glucose response to food. If you have a treat—ice cream on a hot summer's day or delicious pizza—watch your glucose response.

When you're insulin resistant, your blood sugar will shoot up sky-high and it will stay sky-high for hours. If you have reversed your type 2 diabetes, your blood sugar will go up in response to the insulin surge from these treats, but it will return to your baseline within about two hours. That means the body is producing adequate insulin and that you've overcome insulin resistance. Your body is processing glucose as it comes in and returning your blood sugar levels to baseline within two hours or so.

Weight loss

You'll know by stepping on the scale how much you weigh, but the scale can't tell you if you've reset your insulin resistance issues. At least, not right away. What I want you to do is record the number on the scale over several weeks.

Think of your body weight like the temperature in a home. The temperature may increase or decrease but it will return to the temperature you've set on the thermostat. Your body works the same way; its thermostat is our body weight set point, and it's the equilibrium point that our body will return to. Let's say, for example, that your body weight set point is 200 pounds. You go on vacation and eat a lot, have a few days of illness, and then perhaps indulge at a wedding. What you'll find is that your weight may fluctuate up or down day to day, but overall your weight will hover around your body weight set point of 200 pounds.

Through intermittent fasting, your body weight set point will decrease over time. You may see it drop from, say, 200 to 145 pounds. And you may fear that as soon as you indulge—at a holiday celebration or a birthday party, for example—you'll rapidly gain back all the weight you've lost. What I've seen in the clinic, again and again, is that as clients lower this body weight set point, their body naturally returns to that new equilibrium point. Women are so nervous to step on the scale, telling me they've been on vacation and eaten so much, but because their body has healed from insulin resistance and they have a new body weight set point, their weight naturally stays close to the new normal. They have reset the thermostat of their house.

At this point, I want you to stop thinking about your weight altogether. Instead, I want you to start thinking about *fat loss*. When we step on the scale, it doesn't tell us how much fat we have, merely how much mass we have. The scale tells us:

Fat mass + muscle mass + bone mass + water mass = total weight

The key to long-term health is transforming our relationship with our body, and to do this we want to think about our body composition rather than our total weight. I mentioned that when I first began my fasting journey, I lost 60 pounds, and I felt like I'd done a terrific job. I was wearing size 4/5 clothes, and I felt so proud of how much weight I'd lost. But when I saw my wedding photos, which were taken around this time, I thought, *I don't look metabolically healthy.* My body issues in the past had always been about controlling food, not about how I looked, but just to make sure I wasn't seeing myself with a dysmorphic perspective, I put a sticker over my face in one of the photos. I then asked thirty patients if they thought the person in the photo was overweight. All of them said yes! They were seeing the same thing that I was seeing: the person in the photo looked to be about 15 to 20 pounds overweight. This is when I started to think about body composition and understand it better.

A dual-energy x-ray absorptiometry (DEXA) scan is often used to look at bone density, but it can also measure muscle mass and fat. My DEXA scan at that time showed I was 34 percent fat. Even though I'd lost 60 pounds, 34 percent of my total weight was fat! I had less muscle mass than a normal woman in my age group. I continued to fast and lost another 29 pounds, but only a small amount of fat. At 97 pounds and wearing size 5 clothes, 31 percent of my total weight was still body fat. That was at the high end of normal for a woman my age, and it wasn't metabolically healthy.

I realized I had to take the body composition evidence seriously and transform my path. I started to eat more fats, fast more consistently, and do weight training. I gained muscle mass, and I lost fat. At 124 pounds, I had 24 percent body fat and fit into a size 2 dress. I looked healthier, felt healthier, and was healthier, even though I weighed more than I had at my lowest weight.

As you reach your goal weight, I encourage you to put away the scale and go for a DEXA scan. **Your percentage of body fat, not your overall body weight, should be your target for optimal health.** For women under forty, 18 to 29 percent body fat is ideal. For women over forty, between 18 and 35 percent body fat is optimal. As we fast, we activate the sympathetic nervous system and produce counter-regulatory hormones. Our body produces human growth hormone, which helps us to gain muscle mass on our rebuilding (eating) days. Body weight, therefore, is not a good measure of progress: we may gain weight because we are growing our muscles and adding mass there, which is a good thing. We want strong muscles and bones. Fat loss helps us better understand our overall body composition.

Jamala's Story

Jamala was seventy-two when she first came to the clinic. She was carrying a lot of visceral fat, had developed type 2 diabetes, and had weak bones and osteoporosis. I suggested three 36-hour fasts a week to help her lose weight and reverse her type 2 diabetes.

The next time I saw Jamala was six weeks later. Her husband had had a stroke. He needed care and couldn't help around the house, and so Jamala had been too busy to come into the clinic. She had lost a lot of weight. She joked that her arms were looking tight, and she could see muscles from all the physical activity she'd been doing. She said she'd been fasting a lot because she'd been too busy to eat. And I could see her waist size had shrunk so much that her belt was gigantic on her! She laughed as she said, "Sweetheart, I don't fit *any* of my clothes anymore."

I took her measurements. She'd lost six inches from around her waist! That's exceptional fat loss for a woman who is post-menopausal. Then she stepped onto the scale. Jamala's weight was exactly the same as when she first came to the clinic six weeks before. She saw that number and wept and wept. Instead of seeing her incredible progress—gaining lean mass and losing so much fat—she was stuck on the number on the scale. She believed that weighing the same meant nothing had changed.

To help Jamala see her progress, I ordered a DEXA bone mass scan. The results showed that her osteoporosis had reversed because she had gained bone *and* muscle mass through her increased physical activity. We did further tests to show that she had also lost body fat, and Jamala began to realize the crucial difference between weight loss and fat loss. When she saw this evidence on paper, she finally felt proud of her remarkable journey and realized that her health was improving dramatically—even though her total body weight remained the same.

· EXPERT TIP ·

I encourage every client to put away the scale and to look instead at how clothes fit on their body. To track progress this way, you have to pay attention to how your body is changing. That's the start of developing a relationship with your body rather than with your scale.

I had one client who fit into her fourteen-year-old daughter's yoga pants: she'd gone from being very obese and unhealthy to having a new strong body. Her incredible fat-loss journey brought her a lot of physical energy—which she spent biking a lot with her daughter and husband, and that made her muscles and bones stronger. But the scale did not show her a number she wanted to see; it showed weight gain as she did more activity. So, she put her scale on her driveway and drove over it eight times in her SUV. You don't have to drive over your scale (although you can!), but I do suggest you stop using it to measure success.

Instead, track your progress by taking photos on your fat-loss journey. Use your smartphone—or go retro and use an instant camera. You don't have to share your photos with anyone, but if you take a photo every few weeks and compare it to previous ones, you'll see your progress as your body changes.

You'll also see an increase in inches lost, so another way to track progress is to measure everywhere you carry extra weight. Watch this number go down, and use that as a measurement of success.

· WHAT TO KNOW ABOUT BODY COMPOSITION TESTS ·

A body composition scan can be a useful tool to determine how your body is changing as you fast. Magnetic resonance imaging (MRI) is the gold standard, but in Canada you can't pay to have an MRI done for this purpose. A dual-energy x-ray absorptiometry (DEXA) scan is an excellent alternative, which costs between $60 and $100 and takes less than one minute to do. You lie on a table as a small x-ray ring travels the length of your body. The scan shows where fat is located on your body, whether it's good or bad fat, as well as your muscle mass distribution. The test gives some insight into bone mass too. I recommend that you do body composition scans once every six months at most. Use them to keep an eye on your body, understand it well, and adjust your maintenance strategies, but do not focus on them too much. There are two things to keep in mind:

1 **In general, the scan picks up glycogen stores as muscle mass.** This excess sugar is primarily stored in our muscles—our biceps, triceps, quads—and in our liver. If you eat the standard American diet, you will always store glycogen. If you follow a low-carb diet, you'll get rid of all that glycogen. So, if you do a body scan before you start following a low-carb diet and fasting and again after, your second scan will show much less muscle mass. But what has actually changed is your glycogen stores. If you don't know this, you may become alarmed that you've lost all your muscle! If you have nonalcoholic fatty liver disease (NAFLD), wait until it's resolved before getting a scan. Fatty liver is surplus glycogen stored in the liver, and it shows up as a large muscle in your scan. Waiting until you've reversed your fatty liver to get the scan done gives you much more accurate results about your overall body composition.

2 **For the most accurate results, book the scan after two weeks on your normal routine.** Many people book a body composition scan for the day after Christmas or just after a vacation—when they're off their fasting plan, eating high-carb foods, and looking for motivational data to get themselves back into fasting. Remember, that glycogen shows up in the scan as muscle. Poor eating choices before a DEXA scan makes muscles look bigger in the results. Those same "muscles" will look smaller later on, which can be terribly demotivating.

What Type of Fasting Will Maintain My Goal?

I want to finish with some information about fasting to maintain your goals. The journey onward, like any journey, will be tempered with change and surprises, and it won't end for you when this book does. Take time with these last words here, and know that I'm available online to support your continued path to health and well-being.

Once you meet your healing goals, what you do next depends on your lifestyle choices. If, like many people in our culture, you want to return to snacking and grazing, you will need to maintain a three-times-a-week 24-hour fasting strategy for the long term. If you can manage to cut out snacking completely, you can reduce how many times per week you fast.

Recently I was talking with someone at a dinner party about why people are driven to eat all the time. Her theory was that during hunter-gatherer times, we learned to constantly graze so we wouldn't starve in times of scarcity. I pointed out that we didn't always have access to fresh water, yet we don't frantically drink water all the time. In the same way, we're not designed to eat constantly—it's absolutely against our body's hormonal drive. I truly believe that **cutting out snacking forever is the easiest way**

to stay healthy and maintain fat loss. Beyond cutting out snacks, here are some strategies to maintain success.

Shorter maintenance fasts

When you've reached your immediate healing goals, you can do shorter fasts so long as you don't go back to eating all day long every day.

TIME-RESTRICTED EATING

Most of my clients like to follow a whole food diet with a 14-, 16-, or 18-hour break between their meals every day. This time-restricted eating isn't therapeutic intermittent fasting, but it does minimize the number of times a day that insulin is introduced to the body, which is good for maintenance. I recommend making these breaks intermittent, maybe 14 hours one day, and 16 hours the next day.

Just as nature ebbs and flows, our bodies do best when we change up our routines. You may have experienced this at the gym or with your skincare products—varying the intensity or length of our workout or the type of product we use on our skin can build resilience and adaptability. I believe that fasting and eating work the same way. Be mindful of how you are feeling, how your clothes fit, how your energy levels are. Maybe in the summer when you're sweating and active, you need to eat more. Maybe in the winter when we tend to sit more, we need to fast a bit more.

WEEKLY 24-HOUR FASTS

If you eat more processed and refined foods—maybe because you have kids who like them, and you appreciate the convenience after a busy day of work—I suggest one to two 24-hour fasts a week. Start with one and see how that goes. For the rest of the week, eat normally, perhaps keeping a time-restricted eating habit. After a couple of months, assess how you feel and if your body has remained at its ideal body weight set point. If one 24-hour fast a week isn't enough for you, try two.

ONE MEAL A DAY (OMAD)

A lot of women ask about OMAD because it's easy to fit into their schedule. Although it can work for some women, it's not my preferred option for most clients over the long term. I advise this course of action only if women have a good variety of nutrients in their diet. Micronutrients are very important for our overall health, and OMAD can lead to nutrient deficiencies because it's challenging to eat a wide enough range of foods in one meal. I have seen clients gain weight following this plan because of nutrient deficiencies and slowing metabolism (page 167).

Occasional longer fasts

If a period of eating a lot has caused fat gain, your energy is low, or you want to do a hormonal reset, a longer fast can be helpful. For example, a client in the maintenance stage of fasting was going to Italy for three weeks and wanted to indulge in delicious carb-heavy Italian foods. My advice was to enjoy her holiday and return to her therapeutic fasting protocol (two 48-hour fasts a week) for four to six weeks afterward. Another client lost her best friend suddenly and ate a lot to cope with her grief. She gained a lot of fat. She is trying longer fasts to lose fat and get back to her healthier body.

Longer fasts can also help with disease control. I do an extended fast of five to seven days four times a year because I travel a lot, which upsets my hormonal balance. As I explained in Chapter 10, I think of these longer fasts as part of my annual maintenance program; they're a seasonal cleaning to get rid of junk in my body. For example, the steak I eat at a restaurant might not be as high quality as what I would prepare at home, and it might cause some inflammation in my body. Or it might be dressed in a sauce loaded with sugar, which causes my insulin levels to surge. To counteract these effects, my occasional longer fasts induce autophagy and keep me on my wellness journey. They can be just as helpful for busy women juggling kids, work, and other commitments.

The advice and fasting protocols I recommend for each woman are individualized. I encourage you to try different fasting protocols and learn about your own body: when you're satiated, when you're stressed, and when you need to change your eating because you've attained a new goal. Working with a trusted healthcare practitioner who understands the benefits of fasting (page 18) will strengthen your experience and help you achieve your health goals. Remember, too, that I'm constantly updating information on our website.

What Type of Food Will Maintain My Goal?

Many women come to fasting to lose weight, but they find as they lose fat that they also feel better and really thrive. Women who never wanted to be physically active suddenly crave activity and exercise. They want to optimize their health and well-being for longevity. If you're at this part of your journey, make sure you enjoy it: look at the view, and be proud of everything you've achieved. At the same time, as we become more active, it's crucial to reassess our nutritional demands. Try not to be anxious about that: you don't need to do anything wildly different. To stay in this glorious maintenance mode is not as difficult as most of my clients anticipate it will be.

Eat more natural fats and proteins

A 16/8 fast most days might be the best way to support your nutritional needs and make sure you eat enough . As you become more active, you may become hungrier. I don't recommend eating more frequently throughout the day. Instead, I suggest eating more fats and more proteins. Adding 20 to 30 grams of fat and protein—a couple of ounces of meat, fish, or olive oil—can keep you feeling well and not craving unhealthy foods. If you have brain fog or feel hungry as your activity increases, use the ninety-minute eating strategy (page 210) to establish what fuel your body needs.

Keep your electrolytes up

Don't forget to add that pinch of salt in the morning and to salt your foods, and make sure you add magnesium—with food, as a supplement, or by soaking in Epsom salts. As we heal, we need more of these electrolytes because we don't retain them as well as we used to when we had insulin resistance.

Jenny's Story

Jenny is young and very active, but she has mild PCOS and often carries extra weight. Although Jenny has successfully fasted several times, she struggles with maintaining her healthy lifestyle once she has reached her goal weight. Jenny can easily drop 30 pounds in three months, but then she goes back to her old way of living and regains the weight quickly.

I advised her to continue fasting and using her healthy eating strategies *until she becomes resilient*. It's important to remember that we're trying to heal our cellular selves. Although we might reach our goal weight in a few months and achieve a healthier body composition in twelve to eighteen months, it can take longer to heal our insulin resistance. It is tempting to go back to unhealthy ways of eating once we lose weight, but Jenny must fully heal her body before she can relax her therapeutic eating and fasting protocols. I encourage her to set a new healing goal when she loses the weight, so she doesn't fall back into old habits and perpetuate the cycle.

Jenny's goals continue to evolve. Clients often come to me wanting to get off medication, and then they wish to reverse disease or lose weight. Later in their healing journey, they may want to optimize their body composition. Each part of the journey involves setting new goals as old ones are achieved.

Following a step-by-step approach, Jenny will learn to maintain her health in the long term. She may make a few more mistakes along the way, and she may fall back into her old habits a few more times. But, just like many of my other clients and like me, she'll keep progressing. We don't have to be perfect to progress!

Staying in Your Fasting Journey

To avoid falling into old habits, once you reach your goal, live for a couple of extra months as if you're still trying to reach that goal. That means following your fasting strategy and your nutritional plan. You'll heal cellularly and cement new habits when you give yourself more time to get used to your new ways of eating.

In my journey, I've reached some incredible goals. After six months of therapeutic fasting, I reversed PCOS and type 2 diabetes and I lost fat. But after that, I was so scared to go back to poor health that I continued to follow my fasting strategy for six more months. The results surprised me: I continued to heal emotionally and metabolically, and I improved my relationship with food and my body. I see clients all the time who find that they are more energetic and stronger, and lead happier lives, by continuing to fast for a little longer, even after they've met their original healing goals.

I don't recommend banning foods entirely because that can cause a rebellious thought pattern, but we do want to make treats special. Yes, you should be able to eat pizza or ice cream occasionally and enjoy a slice of cake at a celebration. Your body should become resilient to these treats. But try to stick with your goals to eat healthily most of the time and to keep fasting integrated in your life.

Author Melissa Urban coined the term *food freedom* to describe the idea of being in control of the food that you eat.[1] What she means is that you choose foods you love when it's worth it, skip them when it's not, and don't feel guilty or ashamed for doing either. I like to apply this concept when I'm faced with a treat. I don't eat treats every day, but when I do have them, I really savor them! When I choose to eat pizza, I choose the most delicious, best-quality pizza and enjoy it. I pass on the poor quality choices so that I can enjoy wonderful food. This is what I recommend for you. Set new boundaries so you can incorporate foods you enjoy: you might have ice cream two or three times a year—and when you do, make sure it's the best, most delicious, and most enjoyable experience. Try, too, to stop thinking of these foods as rewards. Like other food, they are fuel and not a reward.

Continue to track your glucose levels to see how different foods impact you. Assess, reassess, incorporate special foods at celebratory times, use the strategies I've shared with you, and slowly transform your relationship with food.

Final Words: Progress, Not Perfection

I hope you've found this book to be everything you've needed. Throughout these pages, I've followed the approach I follow with my clients. I treat everyone I work with as an individual, and I love to help them find their own path to wellness. Hopefully this book has helped you find your own path, and may your journey be wonderful.

Wellness *is* a journey, and that means you need to keep in mind that every step is about progress, not perfection. Remember not to get discouraged if you take a wrong turn or you feel you're not progressing fast enough. Not everyone's journey is linear. I believe the saying "It's never a failure and always a lesson" so much that I have those words inked on my body.

I also truly believe that if I can do this, then anyone can. I'm on this journey with you. There was a time when the woman at the McDonald's drive-thru near the clinic called me "Babydoll" and knew my order because I was there so often. I ate poorly and was very unhealthy. If I can change my relationship with food— now I crave a cup of tea when I'm stressed instead of a bag of pretzels—then you can too. The secret to success is to take small, consistent steps and accept that you'll make mistakes along the way. Instead of aiming for seven days of perfect eating, I learned to aim for eating healthy food one day a week, and slowly I learned how to fast. Slow and steady worked for me, and it's how I continue to manage my weight and my health. It will work for you.

Remember that you're human and it's okay to make mistakes and break your fast early. Lean on your community for support. Join me and others on their own wellness journeys online in our community. I'm there all the time, learning, sharing, and connecting. Come and share your story, ask a question, and celebrate as we make changes and transform our lives together.

Chapter 13 Takeaways

- It can be challenging to reach our fasting goals and know how to measure success. Gauge your progress using qualitative measures (human moments), body composition scans, and photos so that you can really see the results.

- To maintain your healing goals, try to avoid snacking and follow a time-restricted eating plan. If snacking is a regular part of your life, stick with a fasting protocol.

- Occasional fasts can be helpful to return to your body weight set point after eating poorly for a period of time or to prevent disease.

- Remember, it's never a failure and always a lesson. Please don't engage in self-sabotage. You are on a journey and it's about progress, not perfection.

- Be proud of everything you've achieved. And keep learning. You can return to this book as you need to, and connect with me and others online. If I can make these changes, anyone can!

Acknowledgments

I WANT TO THANK my clinic patients. They enabled me to learn how to help so many people through my online platform, and while I was supporting them, they helped to support me. This community helped me thrive. I couldn't have done this on my own.

I thank my online community and community mentors who have become friends. It's been so great to have friends with a similar lifestyle to me. Thanks to my entire team for being there every day. We're connected by our desire to be lifelong students and support one another. We're not just colleagues; we're family.

Thanks to the team at Greystone Books, especially to Lucy Kenward and Rob Sanders for working hard with me to ensure that this book could get out into the world.

I want to thank Dr. Jason Fung for bringing fasting, the original human diet, back to the forefront of public awareness and for fighting all the fights to have us taken seriously. Thanks for saving my life and collaborating with me to save the lives of so many other people. I have always wanted to help people, and conventional medicine wasn't doing all it could. Now I can fulfill my dream of helping people.

Thank you to my mom and my brother, who is also one of my teammates and works tirelessly on the business side to keep us growing.

I couldn't have completed this book without the support of my dear friend Alice. She's a wonderful sounding board and was a source of great emotional support throughout the process.

And most of all, thank you to my husband, Angel, who is incredibly supportive and a true partner in every aspect of our relationship. When I work long hours and long days, he puts his life on hold to help me get my message out there. He believes in me more than anyone. I'm a lucky woman. I look forward to every day of our journey together.

Appendix
Sample Fasting Plans

Three 24-hour fasts a week

DAY 1	DAY 2	DAY 3	DAY 4	DAY 5	DAY 6	DAY 7
FAST	FAST	FAST	FAST	FAST	FAST	FAST
Lunch	FAST	Lunch	FAST	Lunch	FAST	Lunch
Dinner	Dinner	Dinner	Dinner	Dinner	Dinner	Dinner

Three 30-hour fasts a week

DAY 1	DAY 2	DAY 3	DAY 4	DAY 5	DAY 6	DAY 7
Breakfast	FAST	Breakfast	FAST	Breakfast	FAST	Breakfast
Lunch	FAST	Lunch	FAST	Lunch	FAST	Lunch
FAST	Dinner	FAST	Dinner	FAST	Dinner	FAST

Three 36-hour fasts a week

DAY 1	DAY 2	DAY 3	DAY 4	DAY 5	DAY 6	DAY 7
Breakfast	FAST	Breakfast	FAST	Breakfast	FAST	Breakfast
Lunch	FAST	Lunch	FAST	Lunch	FAST	Lunch
Dinner	FAST	Dinner	FAST	Dinner	FAST	Dinner

Three 42-hour fasts a week

DAY 1	DAY 2	DAY 3	DAY 4	DAY 5	DAY 6	DAY 7
FAST	FAST	FAST	FAST	FAST	FAST	FAST
Lunch	FAST	Lunch	FAST	Lunch	FAST	Lunch
Dinner	FAST	Dinner	FAST	Dinner	FAST	Dinner

Two 48-hour fasts a week

DAY 1	DAY 2	DAY 3	DAY 4	DAY 5	DAY 6	DAY 7
FAST	FAST	FAST	FAST	FAST	FAST	FAST
Lunch	FAST	FAST	Lunch	FAST	FAST	Lunch
Dinner	FAST	Dinner	Dinner	FAST	Dinner	Dinner

Two 66-hour fasts a week

DAY 1	DAY 2	DAY 3	DAY 4	DAY 5	DAY 6	DAY 7
FAST	FAST	FAST	FAST	FAST	FAST	FAST
Lunch	FAST	FAST	Lunch	FAST	FAST	Lunch
Dinner	FAST	FAST	Dinner	FAST	FAST	Dinner

One 72-hour fast plus a 24-hour fast each week

DAY 1	DAY 2	DAY 3	DAY 4	DAY 5	DAY 6	DAY 7
FAST	FAST	FAST	FAST	FAST	FAST	FAST
Lunch	FAST	FAST	FAST	Lunch	FAST	Lunch
Dinner	FAST	FAST	Dinner	Dinner	Dinner	Dinner

Notes

1: The Benefits and Myths of Intermittent Fasting for Women

1 Victoria A. Catenacci et al., "A Randomized Pilot Study Comparing Zero-Calorie Alternate-Day Fasting to Daily Caloric Restriction in Adults With Obesity," *Obesity* 24, 9 (2016): 1874–83, https://doi.org/10.1002/oby.21581.

2 Catenacci et al., "A Randomized Pilot Study."

3 Catenacci et al., "A Randomized Pilot Study."

4 A.M. Johnstone et al., "Effect of an Acute Fast on Energy Compensation and Feeding Behaviour in Lean Men and Women," *International Journal of Obesity* 26, 12 (December 2002): 1623–28, https://doi.org/10.1038/sj.ijo.0802151.

2: Calorie Confusion

1 Kevin D. Hall and Scott Kahan, "Maintenance of Lost Weight and Long-Term Management of Obesity," *Medical Clinics of North America* 102, 1 (January 2018): 183–97, https://doi.org/10.1016/j.mcna.2017.08.012.

2 Jordyn Taylor, "Why Do So Many 'Biggest Loser' Contestants Struggle to Keep the Weight Off?" *Yahoo! News*, May 2, 2016, https://sg.news.yahoo.com/why-many-biggest-loser-contestants-201000001.html; Gina Kolata, "After 'The Biggest Loser,' Their Bodies Fought to Regain Weight," *New York Times*, May 2, 2016, https://www.nytimes.com/2016/05/02/health/biggest-loser-weight-loss.html.

3 Leah M. Kalm and Richard D. Semba, "They Starved So That Others Be Better Fed: Remembering Ancel Keys and the Minnesota Experiment," *Journal of Nutrition* 135, 6 (June 2005): 1347–52, https://doi.org/10.1093/jn/135.6.1347.

4 Barbara V. Howard et al., "Low-Fat Dietary Pattern and Weight Change Over 7 Years: The Women's Health Initiative Dietary Modification Trial," *JAMA* 295, 1 (January 2006): 39–49, https://doi.org/10.1001/jama.295.1.39.

5 I-Min Lee et al., "Physical Activity and Weight Gain Prevention," *JAMA* 303, 12 (March 2010): 1173–79, https://doi.org/10.1001/jama.2010.312.

6 John Cloud, "Why Exercise Won't Make You Thin," *Time*, August 9, 2009, https://content.time.com/time/subscriber/article/0,33009,1914974,00.html.

7 Diabetes Prevention Program Research Group et al., "10-Year Follow-Up of Diabetes Incidence and Weight Loss in the Diabetes Prevention Program Outcomes Study," *Lancet* 374, 9702 (November 2009): 1677–86, https://doi.org/10.1016/s0140-6736(09)61457-4.

8   Look AHEAD Research Group et al., "The Look AHEAD Study: A Description of the Lifestyle Intervention and the Evidence Supporting It," *Obesity* 14, 5 (May 2006): 737-52, https://doi.org/10.1038/oby.2006.84.

9   The HEALTHY Study Group, "A School-Based Intervention for Diabetes Risk Reduction," *New England Journal of Medicine* 363 (July 2010): 443-53, https://doi.org/10.1056/NEJMoa1001933.

10   Peter Boersma, Lindsey I. Black, and Brian W. Ward, "Prevalence of Multiple Chronic Conditions Among US Adults," *Preventing Chronic Disease* 17 (September 2020): 200130, https://doi.org/10.5888/pcd17.200130.

11   "Overweight & Obesity Statistics," National Institute of Diabetes and Digestive and Kidney Diseases, September 2021, https://www.niddk.nih.gov/health-information/health-statistics/overweight-obesity.

12   Kevin D. Hall and Scott Kahan, "Maintenance of Lost Weight and Long-Term Management of Obesity," *Medical Clinics of North America* 102, 1 (January 2018): 183-97, https://doi.org/10.1016/j.mcna.2017.08.012.

13   Rebecca Stamp, "Average Person Will Try 126 Fad Diets in Their Lifetime, Poll Claims," *Independent*, January 8, 2020, https://www.independent.co.uk/life-style/diet-weight-loss-food-unhealthy-eating-habits-a9274676.html.

3: The Role of Insulin Resistance in Obesity and Poor Metabolic Health

1   Hilary A. Coller, "Is Cancer a Metabolic Disease?" *American Journal of Pathology* 184, 1 (January 2014): 4-17, https://doi.org/10.1016/j.ajpath.2013.07.035.

4: How a Low-Carb, High-Fat Diet and Fasting Can Transform Your Health

1   Christian Zauner et al., "Resting Energy Expenditure in Short-Term Starvation Is Increased as a Result of an Increase in Serum Norepinephrine," *American Journal of Clinical Nutrition* 71, 6 (June 2000): 1511-15, https://doi.org/10.1093/ajcn/71.6.1511.

2   Sayed Hossein Davoodi et al., "Calorie Shifting Diet Versus Calorie Restriction Diet: A Comparative Clinical Trial Study," *International Journal of Preventive Medicine* 5, 4 (April 2014): 447-56, https://www.ncbi.nlm.nih.gov/pmc/articles/PMC4018593.

3   Victoria A. Catenacci et al., "A Randomized Pilot Study Comparing Zero-Calorie Alternate-Day Fasting to Daily Caloric Restriction in Adults With Obesity," *Obesity* 24, 9 (2016): 1874-83, https://doi.org/10.1002/oby.21581.

4   Corey A. Rynders et al., "Effectiveness of Intermittent Fasting and Time-Restricted Feeding Compared to Continuous Energy Restriction for Weight Loss," *Nutrients* 11, 10 (October 2019): 2442, https://doi.org/10.3390/nu11102442.

5: Cortisol

1   Judith A. Whitworth et al., "Hyperinsulinemia Is Not a Cause of Cortisol-Induced Hypertension," *American Journal of Hypertension* 7, 6 (June 1994): 562-65, https://doi.org/10.1093/ajh/7.6.562.

2   G. Pagano et al., "An In Vivo and In Vitro Study of the Mechanism of Prednisone-Induced Insulin Resistance in Healthy Subjects," *Journal of Clinical Investigation* 72, 5 (November 1983): 1814-20, https://doi.org/10.1172/JCI111141.

3   Robert A. Rizza, Lawrence J. Mandarino, and John E. Gerich, "Cortisol-Induced Insulin Resistance in Man: Impaired Suppression of Glucose Production and Stimulation of Glucose Utilization due to a Postreceptor Detect of Insulin Action," *Journal of Clinical Endocrinology & Metabolism* 54, 1 (January 1982): 131–38, https://doi.org/10.1210/jcem-54-1-131.

4   R.P. Stolk et al., "Gender Differences in the Associations Between Cortisol and Insulin in Healthy Subjects," *Journal of Endocrinology* 149, 2 (May 1996): 313–18, https://doi.org/10.1677/joe.0.1490313.

5   R.M. Jindal, "Posttransplant Diabetes Mellitus—A Review," *Transplantation* 58, 12 (December 1994): 1289–98, https://pubmed.ncbi.nlm.nih.gov/7809919.

6   Rizza, Mandarino, and Gerich, "Cortisol-Induced Insulin Resistance in Man."

7   Isabelle Lemieux et al., "Effects of Prednisone Withdrawal on the New Metabolic Triad in Cyclosporine-Treated Kidney Transplant Patients," *Kidney International* 62, 5 (November 2002): 1839–47, https://doi.org/10.1046/j.1523-1755.2002.00611.x.

8   Mattia Barbot, Filippo Ceccato, and Carla Scaroni, "Diabetes Mellitus Seconary to Cushing's Disease," *Frontiers in Endocrinology* 9 (June 2018), https://doi.org/10.3389/fendo.2018.00284.

9   Hammad S. Chaudhry and Gurdeep Singh, "Cushing Syndrome," StatPearls, June 27, 2022, https://www.ncbi.nlm.nih.gov/books/NBK470218/.

10   Robert Fraser et al., "Cortisol Effects on Body Mass, Blood Pressure, and Cholesterol in the General Population," *Hypertension* 33, 6 (June 1999): 1364–68, https://doi.org/10.1161/01.hyp.33.6.1364.

11   *Your Guide to Healthy Sleep*, US Department of Health and Human Services and National Heart, Lung, and Blood Institute, August 2011, www.nhlbi.nih.gov/files/docs/public/sleep/healthy_sleep.pdf.

12   Eun Yeon Joo et al., "Adverse Effects of 24 Hours of Sleep Deprivation on Cognition and Stress Hormones," *Journal of Clinical Neurology* 8, 2 (June 2012): 146–50, https://doi.org/10.3988/jcn.2012.8.2.146.

13   Gregor Hasler et al., "The Association Between Short Sleep Duration and Obesity in Young Adults: A 13-Year Prospective Study," *Sleep* 27, 4 (June 2004): 661–66, https://doi.org/10.1093/sleep/27.4.661.

14   Jun Wang and Xin Ren, "Association Between Sleep Duration and Sleep Disorder Data From the National Health and Nutrition Examination Survey and Stroke Among Adults in the United States," *Medical Science Monitor* 28 (July 2022), e936384, https://doi.org/10.12659/MSM.936384; Chloe M. Beverly Hery, Lauren Hale, and Michelle J. Naughton, "Contributions of the Women's Health Initiative to Understanding Associations Between Sleep Duration, Insomnia Symptoms, and Sleep-Disordered Breathing Across a Range of Health Outcomes in Postmenopausal Women," *Sleep Health* 6, 1 (February 2020): 48–59, https://doi.org/10.1016/j.sleh.2019.09.005; *Your Guide to Healthy Sleep*.

15 Jean-Philippe Chaput et al., "The Association Between Sleep Duration and Weight Gain in Adults: A 6-Year Prospective Study From the Quebec Family Study," *Sleep* 31, 4 (April 2008): 517–23, https://doi.org/10.1093/sleep/31.4.517.

16 Hasler et al., "The Association Between Short Sleep Duration and Obesity in Young Adults."

17 Mayumi Watanabe et al., "Association of Short Sleep Duration With Weight Gain and Obesity at 1-Year Follow-Up: A Large-Scale Prospective Study," *Sleep* 33, 2 (February 2010): 161–67, https://doi.org/10.1093/sleep/33.2.161.

18 Francesco P. Cappuccio et al., "Meta-Analysis of Short Sleep Duration and Obesity in Children and Adults," *Sleep* 31, 5 (May 2008): 619–26, https://doi.org/10.1093/sleep/31.5.619.

19 Lisa Rafalson et al., "Short Sleep Duration Is Associated With the Development of Impaired Fasting Glucose: The Western New York Health Study," *Annals of Epidemiology* 20, 12 (December 2010): 883–89, https://doi.org/10.1016/j.annepidem.2010.05.002.

20 Rachel Leproult et al., "Sleep Loss Results in an Elevation of Cortisol Levels the Next Evening," *Sleep* 20, 10 (October 1997): 865–70, https://doi.org/10.1093/sleep/20.10.865.

21 Lisa Morselli et al., "Role of Sleep Duration in the Regulation of Glucose Metabolism and Appetite," *Best Practice & Research Clinical Endocrinology & Metabolism* 24, 5 (October 2010): 687–702, https://doi.org/10.1016/j.beem.2010.07.005.

22 Karine Spiegel et al., "Sleep Loss: A Novel Risk Factor for Insulin Resistance and Type 2 Diabetes," *Journal of Applied Physiology* 99, 5 (November 2005): 2008–19, https://doi.org/10.1152/japplphysiol.00660.2005.

23 Norito Kawakami, Naoyoshi Takatsuka, and Hiroyuki Shimizu, "Sleep Disturbance and Onset of Type 2 Diabetes," *Diabetes Care* 27, 1 (January 2004): 282–83, https://doi.org/10.2337/diacare.27.1.282.

24 Chaput et al., "The Association Between Sleep Duration and Weight Gain in Adults."

25 Slobodanka Pejovic et al., "Leptin and Hunger Levels in Young Healthy Adults After One Night of Sleep Loss," *Journal of Sleep Research* 19, 4 (December 2010): 552–58, https://doi.org/10.1111/j.1365-2869.2010.00844.x.

26 Young Kyung Do, "The Effect of Sleep Duration on Body Weight in Adolescents," Stanford Asia Health Policy Program Working Paper 38, February 2014, https://ssrn.com/abstract=2393704.

27 Jennifer Daubenmier et al., "Mindfulness Intervention for Stress Eating to Reduce Cortisol and Abdominal Fat Among Overweight and Obese Women: An Exploratory Randomized Controlled Study," *Journal of Obesity* 2011 (2011): 651936, https://doi.org/10.1155/2011/651936.

28 Jennifer Daubenmier et al., "It's Not What You Think, It's How You Relate to It," *Psychoneuroendocrinology* 48 (October 2014): 11–18, https://doi.org/10.1016/j.psyneuen.2014.05.012.

6: How Estrogen Dominance Disrupts Menstruation and Metabolism

1 Angelo Cagnacci and Martina Venier, "The Controversial History of Hormone Replacement Therapy," *Medicina* 55, 9 (September 2019): 602, https://doi.org/10.3390/medicina55090602.

7: How Too Much Insulin Can Lead to Elevated Testosterone and Polycystic Ovary Syndrome

1   "History of Discovery of Polycystic Ovary Syndrome," *Advances in Clinical and Experimental Medicine* 26, 3 (May–June 2017): 555–58, https://doi.org/10.17219/acem/61987.

2   For example, Ewa Otto-Buczkowska, Karolina Grzyb, and Natalia Jainta, "Polycystic Ovary Syndrome (PCOS) and the Accompanying Disorders of Glucose Homeostasis Among Girls at the Time of Puberty," *Pediatric Endocrinology Diabetes and Metabolism* 24, 1 (2018): 40–44, https://doi.org/10.18544/PEDM-24.01.0101; P. Moghetti and F. Tosi, "Insulin Resistance and PCOS: Chicken or Egg?" *Journal of Endocrinological Investigation* 44 (February 2021): 233–44, https://doi.org/10.1007/s40618-020-01351-0.

3   Maria-Elisabeth Smet and Andrew McLennan, "Rotterdam Criteria, the End," *Australasian Journal of Ultrasound in Medicine* 21, 2 (May 2018): 59–60, https://doi.org/10.1002/ajum.12096.

4   Ricardo Azziz et al., "Health Care-Related Economic Burden of the Polycystic Ovary Syndrome During the Reproductive Life Span," *Journal of Clinical Endocrinology & Metabolism* 90, 8 (August 2005): 4650–58, https://doi.org/10.1210/jc.2005-0628.

5   Sydney Parker, "When Missed Periods Are a Metabolic Problem," *The Atlantic*, June 25, 2015, https://www.theatlantic.com/health/archive/2015/06/polycystic-ovary-syndrome-pcos/396116.

6   Roger Hart et al., "Definitions, Prevalence and Symptoms of Polycystic Ovaries and Polycystic Ovary Syndrome," *Best Practice & Research Clinical Obstetrics & Gynaecology* 18, 5 (October 2004): 671–83, https://doi.org/10.1016/j.bpobgyn.2004.05.001.

7   Pratip Chakraborty et al., "Recurrent Pregnancy Loss in Polycystic Ovary Syndrome: Role of Hyperhomocysteinemia and Insulin Resistance," *PLOS ONE* 8, 5 (May 2013): e64446, https://doi.org/10.1371/journal.pone.0064446.

8   Anju E. Joham et al., "Prevalence of Infertility and Use of Fertility Treatment in Women With Polycystic Ovary Syndrome: Data From a Large Community-Based Cohort Study," *Journal of Women's Health* 24, 4 (April 2015): 299–307, http://doi.org/10.1089/jwh.2014.5000.

9   Enrico Carmina and Rogerio A. Lobo, "Polycystic Ovary Syndrome (PCOS): Arguably the Most Common Endocrinopathy Is Associated With Significant Morbidity in Women," *Journal of Clinical Endocrinology & Metabolism* 84, 6 (June 1999): 1897–99, https://doi.org/10.1210/jcem.84.6.5803; Adam H. Balen et al., "Miscarriage Rates Following In-Vitro Fertilization Are Increased in Women With Polycystic Ovaries and Reduced by Pituitary Desensitization With Buserelin," *Human Reproduction* 8, 6 (June 1993): 959–64, https://doi.org/10.1093/oxfordjournals.humrep.a138174.

10 C.M. Boomsma et al., "A Meta-Analysis of Pregnancy Outcomes in Women With Polycystic Ovary Syndrome," *Human Reproduction Update* 12, 6 (November/December 2006): 673–83, https://doi.org/10.1093/humupd/dml036.

11 Patrick M. Catalano et al., "Gestational Diabetes and Insulin Resistance: Role in Short- and Long-Term Implications for Mother and Fetus," *Journal of Nutrition* 133, 5 (May 2003): 1674S–83S, https://doi.org/10.1093/jn/133.5.1674S.

12 Boomsma et al., "A Meta-Analysis of Pregnancy Outcomes."

13 Bradley G. Chittenden et al., "Polycystic Ovary Syndrome and the Risk of Gynae-cological Cancer: A Systematic Review," *Reproductive Biomedicine Online* 19, 3 (September 2009): 398–405, https://doi.org/10.1016/s1472-6483(10)60175-7.

14 "Cancers Associated With Overweight and Obesity Make Up 40 Percent of Cancers Diagnosed in the United States," Centers for Disease Control and Prevention, press release, October 3, 2017, https://www.cdc.gov/media/releases/2017/p1003-vs-cancer-obesity.html.

15 E. Dahlgren et al., "Polycystic Ovary Syndrome and Risk for Myocardial Infarction," *Acta Obstetricia et Gynecologica Scandinavica* 71, 8 (December 1992): 599–604, https://doi.org/10.3109/00016349209006227.

16 Carmina and Lobo, "Polycystic Ovary Syndrome (PCOS)"; Natalie L. Rasgon et al., "Reproductive Function and Risk for PCOS in Women Treated for Bipolar Disorder," *Bipolar Disorders* 7, 3 (June 2005): 246–59, https://doi.org/10.1111/j.1399-5618 .2005.00201.x.

17 Heather R. Peppard et al., "Prevalence of Polycystic Ovary Syndrome Among Premenopausal Women With Type 2 Diabetes," *Diabetes Care* 24, 6 (June 2001): 1050–52, https://doi.org/10.2337/diacare.24.6.1050.

18 Evanthia Diamanti-Kandarakis and Andrea Dunaif, "Insulin Resistance and the Polycystic Ovary Syndrome Revisited," *Endocrine Reviews* 33, 6 (December 2012): 981-1030, https://doi.org/10.1210/er.2011-1034.

19 Ethel Codner et al., "Diagnostic Criteria for Polycystic Ovary Syndrome and Ovar-ian Morphology in Women With Type 1 Diabetes Mellitus," *Journal of Clinical Endocrinology & Metabolism* 91, 6 (June 2006): 2250–56, https://doi.org/10.1210/ jc.2006-0108.

20 Carly E. Kelley et al., "Review of Nonalcoholic Fatty Liver Disease in Women With Polycystic Ovary Syndrome," *World Journal of Gastroenterology* 20, 39 (October 2014): 14172–84, https://doi.org/10.3748/wjg.v20.i39.14172.

21 A.L.L. Rocha et al., "Non-Alcoholic Fatty Liver Disease in Women With Polycystic Ovary Syndrome," *Journal of Endocrinological Investigation* 40, 12 (December 2017): 1279–88, https://doi.org/10.1007/s40618-017-0708-9.

22 Evangeline Vassilatou, "Nonalcoholic Fatty Liver Disease and Polycystic Ovary Syndrome," *World Journal of Gastroenterology* 20, 26 (July 2014): 8351–63, https:// doi.org/10.3748/wjg.v20.i26.8351; Kelley et al., "Review of Nonalcoholic Fatty Liver Disease."

23 Alexandros N. Vgontzas et al., "Polycystic Ovary Syndrome Is Associated With Obstructive Sleep Apnea and Daytime Sleepiness," *Journal of Clinical Endocri-nology & Metabolism* 86, 2 (February 2001): 517–20, https://doi.org/10.1210/ jcem.86.2.7185; Balachandran Kumarendran et al., "Increased Risk of Obstructive Sleep Apnoea in Women With Polycystic Ovary Syndrome," *European Journal of Endocrinology* 180, 4 (April 2019): 265–72, https://doi.org/10.1530/EJE-18-0693.

24 R.D. Murray et al., "Clinical Presentation of PCOS Following Development of an Insulinoma: Case Report," *Human Reproduction* 15, 1 (January 2000): 86–88, https://doi.org/10.1093/humrep/15.1.86.

25 D. Micic et al., "Androgen Levels During Sequential Insulin Euglycemic Clamp Studies in Patients With Polycystic Ovary Disease," *Journal of Steroid Biochemistry* 31, 6 (December 1988): 995–99, https://doi.org/10.1016/0022-4731(88)90344-5.

26 Stephen Franks et al., "Etiology of Anovulation in Polycystic Ovary Syndrome," *Steroids* 63, 5–6 (May–June 1998): 306–7, https://doi.org/10.1016/s0039-128x(98)00035-x; Sophie Jonard and Didier Dewailly, "The Follicular Excess in Polycystic Ovaries, Due to Intra-Ovarian Hyperandrogenism, May Be the Main Culprit for the Follicular Arrest," *Human Reproduction Update* 10, 2 (March–April 2004): 107–17, https://doi.org/10.1093/humupd/dmh010.

9: How to Begin and Extend Shorter Fasts

1 Dylan A. Lowe et al., "Effects of Time-Restricted Eating on Weight Loss and Other Metabolic Parameters in Women and Men With Overweight and Obesity," *JAMA Internal Medicine* 180, 11 (September 2020): 1491–99, https://doi.org/10.1001/jamainternmed.2020.4153; Deying Liu et al., "Calorie Restriction With or Without Time-Restricted Eating in Weight Loss," *New England Journal of Medicine* 386 (April 2022): 1495–504, https://doi.org/10.1056/NEJMoa2114833.

11: Tips and Tricks for Troubleshooting Fasts

1 Mario Barbagallo and Ligia J. Dominguez, "Magnesium and Type 2 Diabetes," *World Journal of Diabetes* 6, 10 (August 2015): 1152–57, https://doi.org/10.4239/wjd.v6.i10.1152; Debora Porri et al., "Effect of Magnesium Supplementation on Women's Health and Well-Being," *NFS Journal* 23 (June 2021): 30–36, https://doi.org/10.1016/j.nfs.2021.03.003.

2 Pradeep M.K. Nair and Pranav G. Khawale, "Role of Therapeutic Fasting in Women's Health: An Overview," *Journal of Mid-Life Health* 7, 2 (April–June 2016): 61–64, https://doi.org/10.4103/0976-7800.185325.

12: Tips and Tricks for Building a Healthy Relationship With Food

1 Lily Nichols, "CGM Experiment: Part 2—A Tale of Two Breakfasts," LilyNicholsRDN.com, n.d., https://lilynicholsrdn.com/cgm-experiment-part-2/.

2 Rebecca Stamp, "Average Person Will Try 126 Fad Diets in Their Lifetime, Poll Claims," *Independent*, January 8, 2020, https://www.independent.co.uk/life-style/diet-weight-loss-food-unhealthy-eating-habits-a9274676.html.

13: How to Make Fasting and Healthy Eating a Lifelong Habit

1 Melissa Urban, "What Is Food Freedom?" Whole30.com, February 26, 2021, https://whole30.com/what-is-food-freedom.

Index

Note: Page references in italics indicate figures or illustrations